Baillière's Study Skills for Nurses and Midwives

For Baillière Tindall:
Senior Commissioning Editor: Ninette Premdas
Project Development Editor: Katrina Mather
Project Manager: Andrew Palfreyman
Design: George Ajayi

Baillière's Study Skills for Nurses and Midwives

Third Edition

Edited by

Sian Maslin-Prothero
Professor of Nursing, Keele University, Keele, UK

Foreword by

Bob Price
Programme Director, MSc in Nursing, Lecturer in Distance
Learning, RCN Institute, London, UK

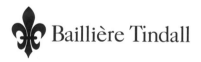 Baillière Tindall

EDINBURGH LONDON NEW YORK OXFORD PHILADELPHIA ST LOUIS SYDNEY TORONTO 2005

BAILLIÈRE TINDALL
An imprint of Elsevier Limited

© Baillière Tindall 1997
© Harcourt Publishers Limited 2001
© Elsevier Science Limited 2002
© Elsevier Science Limited 2005. All rights reserved.

List publication years of previous editions:
First edition 1997
Second edition 2001
Third edition 2005

ISBN 0 70202766 9

British Library Cataloguing in Publication Data
A catalogue record for this book is available from the British Library

Library of Congress Cataloging in Publication Data
A catalog record for this book is available from the Library of Congress

Note
Medical knowledge is constantly changing. Standard safety precautions must be followed, but as new research and clinical experience broaden our knowledge, changes in treatment and drug therapy may become necessary or appropriate. Readers are advised to check the most current product information provided by the manufacturer of each drug to be administered to verify the recommended dose, the method and duration of administration, and contraindications. It is the responsibility of the practitioner, relying on experience and knowledge of the patient, to determine dosages and the best treatment for each individual patient. Neither the Publisher nor the editor assumes any liability for any injury and/or damage to persons or property arising from this publication.

The Publisher

 ELSEVIER   your source for books, journals and multimedia in the health sciences

www.elsevierhealth.com

The Publisher's policy is to use paper manufactured from sustainable forests

Printed in China

Contents

Contributors

Denis Anthony
Professor of Nursing Informatics, University of De Montfort, Leicester, UK

Sue Brain
Library Services Manager, NHS Direct Hampshire & Isle of Wight and NHS Direct Online, Southampton, UK

Elizabeth A Girot
Principal Lecturer, Faculty of Health and Social Care, University of the West of England, Bristol, UK

Maggie Mallik
Head of Interprofessional Practice Learning, Nottingham Health Community, Nottingham, UK

Kym Martindale
Senior Lecturer, Faculty of Media and Culture, University College Falmouth, Cornwall, UK

Sian Maslin-Prothero
Professor of Nursing, Keele University, Keele, UK

Abigail Masterson
Director, Abi Masterson Consulting Ltd, London, UK

Liz Redfern
Director of Patient Care & Nursing Services, Taunton & Somerset Hospital, Taunton, UK

Ian Welsh
Principal Lecturer, Nursing & Healthcare Studies, John Moores University, Liverpool, UK

Heather Wharrad
Senior Lecturer, School of Nursing, University of Nottingham, Nottingham, UK

And sadly, **Anne Palmer** (formerly of the Department of Community and Collaborative Practice, University of Westminster, London) who died 9 February 2003.

Foreword

I smile rather ruefully when academic colleagues within Higher Education point out that students attending university should have the requisite study skills to succeed on a course. At one level this view seems naïve, at another not quite up-to-date. Is it really the case that learners acquire the skills of study and thought, simply through association with tutors and peers in the lecture theatre? Isn't it really the case that studying and writing are craft skills that deserve greater attention? I wonder where such colleagues think that students have developed the complex array of skills necessary to achieve a nursing qualification. After all, this is an applied science and a vocational subject – that learned before might not work so well within this setting. It is certainly very easy to forget that within programmes of nurse education there are now a variety of study and academic skills that were not fully exploited in the past. Reflection, critical thinking, the organisation of learning on campus, within the clinical setting and so often through the internet are all features of modern study. In the programme that I lead for instance, students learn to write in seven or eight different ways and each of these requires a degree of scholarship that makes the focus on study skills a priority for students and tutors alike.

There is another good reason for you to pick up and use a book such as this. When you come to university you encounter a different learning and support relationship. The numbers of students taking classes, the requirement for tutors to lecture, research, develop practice and manage administration, make it extremely unlikely that you will secure the intimate environment that we might imagine university entails. Small study groups, in book lined studies are ideal, but they rarely reflect the reality of 21st century higher education. Teaching staff seem more distant somehow and yet they expect so much more of you. The tutor may leave you to arrange personal enquiry or to develop a project and later invite you to engage in discussions on the nature of care or the ethics of practice. It requires an agile and study skills trained mind to get the most from this very adult learning environment. It is much easier to enjoy working with a tutor – the mentor, thought provoker and quizzical companion when you have learned how to study effectively.

This brings us to a brief debate on the best way to learn such study skills. Hopefully, and incrementally, some of these skills you need are learned through interaction with tutors and especially through feed-back on coursework. There is though a strong case to be made for a much more strategic approach to attaining study skills. Alfresco dis-covery can take a long time and prove uncomfortable along the way. It is usually worth investing some time in the conscious planning of study as an activity. Not only will this help you to manage study time better and to enjoy the experience of learning, but it will trigger tech-niques that are just as relevant in nursing practice later on. The well organised and critical thinking student becomes the well prepared prac-titioner of care. Learning to organise study can help you to develop the skills necessary to organise a ward, or plan a new community-based initiative that enriches the lives of others.

With such thoughts in mind then I commend this textbook to your attention. It is the sort of companion that should travel with you throughout your course and which may help provide reassurance when all around seems chaotic. That the recipe of text, activities and reflective points can help students succeed hardly secms in doubt. Students studying distancc learning courses with the RCN Institute and elsewhere have long achieved successful completion rates in excess of 80–90% using just this approach. It therefore seems a wise investment to spend a modest sum on a textbook such as this and an even wiser investment to use this book as you progress through with your own studies. Wherever you live, whatever your university, course or level of experience, I suspect that there will be much to gain by enquiring within.

Bob Price ARRC RGN PhD
Programme Director MSc in Nursing
Professional Lead, Student Support in Distance Learning.

Acknowledgements

I would like to thank Susanne Darra of the University of Wales Swansea for her advice on making this edition applicable to midwifery students.

I would like to thank the contributors to the previous editions of this book, who have provided their knowledge and expertise to make this a very special and different study skills text.

Finally, this book is dedicated to the memory of my mother, Peggy Prothero – one of life's long learners.

Preface

Why learning skills are important

Sian Maslin-Prothero

INTRODUCTION

This preface is an introduction not only to the book but also on being a student of nursing and midwifery. For some of you, it will be read prior to commencing your initial prequalifying course, while others will be undertaking a postqualifying or postgraduate course. For whatever reason, you have decided that through study you will be able to achieve some positive change in your life. Certain practices can assist you as a student to be a successful learner. Even people who have been successful learners in the past, and are confident, can benefit from updating their learning skills.

WHY DO YOU NEED THIS BOOK?

There are a number of reasons why I chose to compile this book; these arose from my experience as a nurse and midwife, as a learner and as a lecturer. The National Health Service (NHS) has evolved and changed since its inception in 1948; and as healthcare professionals we work in an environment of rapid change, where the expectation is that we can respond to these various and changing requirements. This requires strong core skills, and the right 'mind-set' where the individual is able to identify possibilities and solutions, and has the ability to change and adapt to meet new challenges. The introduction of competency-based nursing courses in September 2000 has provided greater access to nurse education for people from a range of backgrounds, including existing NHS staff.

PROFESSIONAL EDUCATION

There is a recognition of the limitations of information and memory and the 'half-life concept' for professional competence, that is the period of time during which half the contents of a course becomes obsolete. What is learned today is only valid for a few years. The estimated half-life for a nursing course is less than 5 years. Through ongoing personal and professional development we can reduce half-life obsolescence. This need for updating ourselves as nurses has been formalized with the introduction of postregistration education and practice (PREP).

Updating our knowledge and skills is now obligatory. To maintain professional registration with the Nursing and Midwifery Council, nurses and midwives must be able to demonstrate that they are competent to practise. This can be demonstrated by completing at least 5 days of study activity during the previous 3 years, and recording this in a personal professional profile (see Chapter 12).

HIGHER EDUCATION

Both pre- and postqualifying education are located in higher education institutions; we have seen nursing and midwifery courses develop from certificate level to diploma and degree level, and beyond to Masters degree and doctoral degree courses. There is an expectation that we have sound knowledge founded on evidence-based practice and learning. This can be achieved through continuing professional development.

WHY LEARNING SKILLS ARE IMPORTANT FOR NURSES AND MIDWIVES

From personal experience I know how important it is to have skills and strategies that can be used when undertaking a course. These will prepare you for the change you experience through study, and identify strategies to help you, not only for this course but also for the rest of your life; such as why do I want to do this course; how will it affect my life; what do I (and others) need to do in order that I get the most from the course? This includes strategies to enable you to successfully achieve your aim of completing any course.

LIFELONG LEARNING SKILLS

There is a need to promote independent activities that foster skills for lifelong learning. As learners you should develop the ability to identify an issue, access and retrieve information, filter it for quality and solve problems. This book aims to equip you with these necessary information-seeking and problem-solving skills, essential for the independent learner.

The English National Board (1995) identifies lifelong learners as being:

- innovative in their practice
- responsive to changing demand
- resourceful in their methods of learning
- able to act as change agents
- able to share good practice and knowledge
- adaptable to changing healthcare needs
- challenging and creative in their practice
- self reliant in their way of working
- responsible and accountable for their work.

These are great expectations. As a nurse lecturer I want to create creative, critical thinkers who can respond to the dynamic health policy environment and the requirements of healthcare consumers, and this book will help you achieve this. As Ferguson (1994, p. 643) stated: 'Learning to learn and learning to practice are essential characteristics of good practice'.

REFERENCES

English National Board 1995 Creating lifelong learners: partnerships for care: guidelines for the implementation of the UKCC's Standards for Education and Practice Following Registration. ENB, London

Ferguson A 1994 Evaluation of the purpose and benefits of continuing education in nursing and the implications for the provision of continuing education for cancer nurses. Journal of Advanced Nursing, 19: 640–646

How to use this book

The book has been divided into three sections. Section I explores the skills required for successful learning, section II examines skills for successful writing and section III looks at learning from practice.

Each chapter consists of a short introduction, as well as a list of key issues to be covered in the chapter. This will allow you to decide quickly whether the chapter contains the information you need. The order in which you read the chapters is entirely up to you. Links to other chapters have been indicated to help you make the most of the book, whatever order you choose.

Above all, the aim of the book is for it to be interactive. The more you attempt the exercises, the more you will get from the book. Keep a notebook near so that you can write down your thoughts. Scribble notes on the book itself (but only if you own it!).

The structure of the chapters has been devised to be as flexible and supportive as possible.

Each chapter begins with

- an introduction
- a list of key issues, letting you know what is covered in the chapter.

WITHIN THE CHAPTER

Case studies

Some chapters contain case studies. These are designed to help you reflect on your own experiences.

Reflection points

These will raise issues that allow you a few moments to reflect on what you are learning and how you might learn from your experiences.

Activities

These invite you as the reader to consider issues that require you to move beyond reflection. They may require you to note down some of your ideas or to carry out some more research into a given topic. You may wish to come back to these after you finish reading the chapter.

Tips and hints

Useful tips have been indicated and highlighted for quick reference. These are often based on the writer's own experiences and we hope they will help you to avoid some of the common pitfalls.

At the end of the chapter, you will usually be asked to reflect on what you have read and how you are going to build on it. More suggestions for further reading and research are sometimes provided too.

1

DEVELOPING YOUR STUDY SKILLS

1 Preparing for your course

Ian Welsh

KEY ISSUES

- ■ Time management
- ■ Setting realistic goals
- ■ Making a timetable
- ■ Making plans
- ■ Defining priorities

- ■ Thinking strategically
  Creating a suitable environment
- ■ Developing networks for support

Preparing for your course

INTRODUCTION

If you have recently started, or are just about to start, a course of study you are also likely to have a high degree of motivation to succeed – whether because of burning ambition or a fear of failure, only you will know. However, congratulate yourself on achieving the first steps to success as a student: the will to succeed and to learn how to study effectively.

One of the things you will realize as you read the chapters in this book is that studying is a serious and time-consuming activity. It is not something to be done as and when you feel like it, like a hobby. Given the commitment you currently have you should aim to maintain your drive and enthusiasm. If you look back on your progress from time to time, you will see what you have achieved and realize that conscientious effort does pay off. This will motivate you to continue.

This first chapter will look at how you can approach studying so that you make the best use of your time and any resources that are available. It will consider timetabling and time management as measures for improving the quality of study time and as strategies for completing important tasks, such as the production of essays and assignments. The final sections will discuss where you study and some of the resources that you may find useful.

The first thing to do is to take a look at yourself, and consider what impact the course is going to have on your life for the foreseeable future. There is no such thing as a 'typical student' and your circumstances may vary considerably from those of your fellow students. If you do not do this you will not be adequately prepared for the demands that the course will make on you; whatever your circumstances you will be required to master the subject matter and demonstrate, through some form of assessment, that you have done so.

PREPARING FOR YOUR COURSE

What best describes your circumstances:

■ Are you a young undergraduate, away from home for the first time?

■ Will you continue to have domestic commitments on top of your study?

■ Will you be taking a part-time course while holding a full-time job (with or without domestic commitments)?

■ Will you need to take a part-time job in order to make ends meet?

■ If it is a taught course, are there likely to be any problems about attending all the lectures and seminars?

■ Can you cope with studying in isolation, if your course is a distance learning one?

Perhaps your circumstances are different from these. Whatever – take some time to think how your life is going to be affected by your new role as a student. What effect is it going to have on others close to you and how will they have to adapt?

Succeeding as a student is a balancing act. You will have to balance your social commitments, personal needs and work obligations against your obligations to yourself as a student. Neglecting any aspect will create an imbalance that may cause you stress and affect the quality of work you submit for assessment.

WHAT IS STUDY?

Before reading any further, take a piece of paper and make a list of the activities that come to mind under the general heading of 'study'.

You may have a list that includes such things as:

■ attending lectures, reading, discussing, essay writing

■ preparing seminars and tutorials, literature searching

■ thinking/reflection

■ clinical skills.

You will see that some of these activities involve working with other students and that some are solitary activities. To do them effectively, you may need to develop new skills, such as how to prepare for seminars or how to read effectively so that you remember what you have read. These aspects are discussed in detail elsewhere in this book. In the meantime, you need to think about the resources you need in order to give yourself the chance to become an effective student.

 Jot down the things that you think you are likely to need to study effectively.

You may have a list that includes such things as:

- time
- a place to study alone
- paper/pens
- books/journals
- access to a library.

Now consider how you could make the most effective use from each of these resources. Remember that this will probably involve obtaining cooperation from partners, children and other people close to you.

PREPARATION

How you learn, where you learn and when you learn will be determined by a number of factors. If you are attending a university you are likely to receive a timetable, which will tell you what to do and where to go at specific times. A timetable will tell you about the times and locations of lectures and seminars. It may also include study time or reading time, which is not linked to a subject. On these occasions you are presented with the opportunity to select 'how' and 'where' you are going to study. A lot of courses are designed on the assumption that you will spend time outside of 'office' hours engaged in activities related to the course. These activities may include:

- reading to support lectures and seminars
- preparation for assignments
- writing essays
- collecting materials for projects.

You may find that these activities conflict with other plans that you have made, such as going out for the evening or watching a film on the television. Making a timetable of your own may help you to avoid or resolve some of these conflicts.

TIME MANAGEMENT

The management of your time, and the activities that fill it, is a very important aspect of studying. When you are studying outside of the time that has been allocated to you in university you will have to make all the decisions. Issues such as 'when' and 'for how long' can be added to 'where' and 'how'. Working at home means mixing your studies into all your other activities. Devoting time to your studies means that you may have less time for some of the other things that you already do. Northedge (1990) identifies three areas that generate activities that are likely to compete for your time: social commitments, work commitments and leisure activities.

■ **Social commitments** include going out to visit friends, time spent with a partner/family, attending parents' evenings or going to church

■ **Work commitments** include housework and childcare as well as attending university and placements (they may also include any agency or part-time work you are engaged in)

■ **Leisure activities** include attending clubs or societies, concerts, sporting activities and going to the pub.

Think about the activities that you are involved in during a typical day.
■ Which activities would you describe as social commitments?
■ Which activities would you describe as work commitments?
■ Which activities would you describe as leisure activities?
■ Which activities take up the most space on your timetable?

If you devote too much time to learning at home, or in university, then your social life and leisure activities will suffer. If you continue to pursue your other commitments without allowing yourself any time for studying it may impede your ability to handle course work or limit your participation in discussions and seminars.

Timetabling will help you to avoid the two extremes. You need to devote some time to studying but it is not desirable to let it take over your life. Keep these two things in mind when you start to make plans:

■ You need to be realistic about what you intend to achieve
■ You need to strike a balance between studying and your other commitments

If you are going to get the most out of the course you will have to be happy and healthy while you study. Studying is not a route to health or happiness, neither is it an effective substitute for them. Remember that you can also learn while you are involved in social or leisure activities with friends, partners or family.

Being realistic will contribute to your sense of wellbeing. If you set yourself demanding goals and then fail to live up to your own expectations, it is possible that you will form a poor impression of your performance. You may end up feeling frustrated and low. If you set an achievable goal you are less likely to fail and more likely to benefit from the pleasant feelings associated with achievement and accomplishment. On the other hand, if the goals you set are easy to achieve, because they are too low, you run the risk of feeling frustrated because you are not making the best of your abilities. You also run the risk of falling behind because you are not doing enough to keep up with the demands of the course.

SETTING REALISTIC GOALS

Setting realistic goals is not a skill that you can put into practice straight away if you are not used to studying. Even people who have learned skills through attending other courses will have to adjust their approach so that it matches the structure and requirements of the current course. Setting goals is a skill that is gained through experience. You may have to learn through trial and error so don't be afraid to experiment and try out all sorts of different things.

- How many hours are you going to work each day?
- Do you prefer to do your work early in the morning or in the evening?
- Do you prefer to arrange set times for breaks (for meals, snacks, drinks, television programmes, etc.) or do you like to work straight through until you have finished?
- Are you going to try and do most of your work during the week so that your weekends are free or are you going to work at weekends so that you can carry on with social and leisure activities throughout the week?

- Try not to get exasperated, upset or angry when you make mistakes
- You can learn from your mistakes as well as your achievements
- Recognize and acknowledge your mistakes

However, it may be helpful to think in relation to long-term, medium-term and short-term goals. For example, at the beginning of a semester you are given a 3000-word essay to be submitted in the last week of semester. Your long-term goal is to write it and submit it on schedule. This does not have to be as daunting as it may appear; if you think about it you may be able to break the task up into smaller components – then ask yourself what sequence they need to be done in. It may be that the first part of the essay involves undertaking a review of the literature – reading what various authors have written on the subject – so clearly that will be your first task, a clearly defined short-term goal. By breaking the major work down like this you will be making it much more manageable, and also less daunting.

Your medium-term goals include

- The production of a draft for part one of the essay after 2 weeks
- An outline of the main points after 4 weeks
- A complete rough draft after 6 weeks.

For each of these there will be a number of tasks to complete (short-term goals). You will need to put time aside to visit the library to borrow books or read journal articles. Don't just assume that it is going to happen, tell yourself that you will do it by a particular date. This approach has the benefit of giving you positive reinforcement. You will see results for your efforts and also feel less daunted by the task; you are in control of it rather than being overwhelmed by it.

MAKING A TIMETABLE

One way of developing a realistic timetable is to work out how much time is available for studying. Make a record of the time you spend in university attending lectures or seminars, as well as of any other work, social commitments and leisure activities that you are engaged in during a typical week. When you know how much of your week is taken up with these activities you will be able to make decisions about the remaining time and how you want (or need) to spend it. Entering the information into a chart like the one shown in Figure 1.1 will help you to create an accurate record.

- How many hours do you spend on work commitments, social commitments and leisure activities each day?
- How are the hours distributed throughout the day?
- Where are the busiest periods?
- Where are the quietest periods?

FIGURE I.I	Time planner

	Mon	Tues	Wed	Thurs	Fri	Sat	Sun
08.00–10.00							
10.00–12.00							
12.00–14.00							
14.00–16.00							
16.00–18.00							
18.00–20.00							
20.00–22.00							

When you have entered all the information that you have collected over a week you will be able to see where the 'free' periods are. The chart will show you where there are chunks of time that are not occupied with leisure, work or social commitments. The chart will also show you if there are clashes between different activities. You will be able to see at a glance if your plan to start something new will involve stopping an existing activity or moving it to another time or day.

This layout has some limitations. These are worth exploring because they are indicative of some of the problems that you are likely to experience whenever you construct schedules of work. The information that has been gathered represents a typical week. If you devise timetables based on the assumption that all the weeks that follow are going to be just like it you may find that your plans are unworkable. Problems may occur because the week that you have chosen to record is not typical. There may be fewer things going on than usual so that the chart has given you a misleading impression of the amount of free time available. Problems will also occur if there is very little repetition in your pattern of activities. If the amount of time you spend on leisure, work and social activities fluctuates, the amount of free time available to you will also fluctuate from week to week. This can make long-term planning difficult.

These limitations do not mean the information that you have collected is useless. It does mean that you need to think about the ways in which it may influence your planning. These suggestions may be useful:

- Be generous when you estimate the amount of time allocated for each activity
- When you recorded different activities did you include time for travelling or changing clothes?
- Did you allocate time for any preparation that has to be done in advance or any tidying that follows an activity?
- Be prepared to adjust your timetable if you do not think it is working

It is better to make changes and modify your expectations than to abandon timetabling or time management altogether. If the timetable that you have made is too tiring or too rigid you could write in more leisure time and reduce your work commitments. If it is too loose and you do not feel that you are making any progress then you may need to develop more structured activities.

MAKING PLANS

Daily, weekly and monthly calendars are useful when you start to make plans. Each calendar can perform a different function:

- monthly calendar – to plan long-range assignments
- weekly calendar – to learn consistency
- daily calendar – to help you set priorities.

From these descriptions you will be able to see that different timescales involve different type of activity.

- *How long is your course? Don't just think about the number of years. Think about the changes that occur during each year. Think about where you will be learning. Where will you be spending most of your time? Will it be on placements or in university? Does this change from year to year?*
- *Where are the significant dates for exams, the submission of essays, clinical placements, etc.? Are certain events or requirements located at the middle or the end of the course? What needs to be done prior to these dates so that you are prepared for them?*
- *Which learning skills do you need to help you prepare for each event? Think about the skills that you have already and then the additional*

skills you will need to learn. Does the programme show you where you will have opportunities to develop these skills? Does the programme show you where you will learn about research, information technology, statistics or drug calculations?

■ *How frequently do you need to check your progress and preparation? This could become more than a checklist of things that you have or have not done. It is your chance to reflect on how things are going. Did you meet your learning outcomes? Were you told what they were or did you negotiate them? Did you enjoy learning? What did you enjoy? Why did you enjoy it? What didn't you like? Why? What do you need to check or make a note of each month? What do you need to check or make a note of each week? What do you need to check or make a note of each day?*

It may help you to think of planning in two stages: long-term and short-term planning. Long-term planning will make you aware of significant dates in the course. These will include assignments, but you will also want to know about holidays, practice placements, study days and reading weeks. All of these will exert some influence over the ways in which you manage your time. Short-term planning may include weekly or daily activities. There may be a clear connection between short-term goals and long-term goals, or you may choose short-term goals to indicate an activity that is carried out regularly. Some goals will show that you want to develop consistency in your study habits while others will show that you are organizing your study time so that you can achieve specific tasks that have been defined as priorities.

Think about all the activities related to learning that you are likely to carry out in the next 2 weeks. Locate each activity on a chart like this so that you can see whether it is more or less urgent, important or not so important.

Important

Urgent   **Not urgent**

Not important

If you put activities near to the important and urgent poles it indicates that you need to think in terms of short-term, rather than long-term, goals. Long-term goals are not always less important. They may indicate something that is ongoing and does not need to be changed or reviewed immediately.

Another useful way of thinking about learning is to make a list of aims and objectives:

■ An aim is a big, broad heading for something you want to achieve. It may involve a piece of work, like the completion of a nursing care assignment, or it may be related to an aspiration such as 'I really want to work on my communication skills during my next placement'.

■ An objective is one of the small steps you have to take in order to achieve your aim. A single aim may incorporate many objectives. Completing an essay will include objectives like carrying out a literature search, writing a plan, writing an introduction, etc. Improving communication skills may involve objectives like using more open questions instead of closed ones, paying close attention to body posture and non-verbal techniques, and improving listening skills.

One of the advantages of sitting down and working out a timetable is that you become more aware of the demands on your time. You will be able to see if there are periods when you will be under a lot of pressure. There may be specific times in the course when you are expected to do two or three things simultaneously. This may involve producing written work for assignment deadlines, changing practice placements or working with mentors and assessors on specific days. In addition, you might also have to complete and submit documentation relating to practice assessments.

Being aware of dates and times will not mean that you can get away with less work but it does encourage you to think about how and when you will get the work done. Your plans may show activities involving family or friends, such as going on holiday, as well as activities related to learning. You will find it useful to look ahead. For example, it is not realistic to set yourself a lot of work during a weekend when you have arranged for a friend to come and stay!

One of the most anxiety-producing situations you can be confronted with is being given a list of submission deadlines and significant dates and not having a strategy for dealing with them. Without a plan you will find it hard to know whether you have done all the things you need to do, or what is the best thing to do next. When people do not have a very clear idea about what needs to be done they may be inclined to procrastinate. This involves avoiding certain jobs or activities because they do not know how to go about them. Procrastination may not produce any short-term discomfort but in the long term it may have serious consequences. The closer you get to a deadline, the greater the pressure. If you avoid an assignment until a week before the submission date you will have to work on it non-stop to meet the deadline.

A task is more easily done if it is not urgent

CASE STUDY

James is in the second month of the Common Foundation programme (CFP). He has been told to do lots of reading and he has a formative essay of 1000 words to write for each of the three sciences represented in the CFP. The essays are not compulsory but he wants to do them because he would like to have some comments on his essay-writing technique. James has not produced any academic work since the end of his course at college 3 years ago and he is worried because he is not sure what the tutors expect from him. He has 6 weeks to write the essays but he also needs to keep up with the reading that has been recommended for the psychology, biology and sociology components of the course.

Put yourself in James' shoes.

■ How would you arrange your study time over the next 6 weeks?

■ How many hours does James need to study if he is going to get the work done?

■ How will that time be divided between producing the essays and keeping up with his reading?

James has stated that he aims to complete three essays within 6 weeks. What are the objectives that will help him to reach this aim?

A nursing course involves different themes or modules, which require separate assessments. It also involves practical work with other nurses and patients or clients. This range of activities means that it is not always possible to drop your other commitments so that you can complete a single task or assignment. If you do drop everything to meet the deadline it may have immediate repercussions on your other commitments. The pressure to meet all of these demands will accumulate and another crisis will develop. If this is the case you are back where you started: under pressure and stressed out!

If you refer to your thoughts about James (in the Case study above) you will recognize that planning involves paying attention to many different aspects of learning. If you are going to reduce your stress levels and avoid rushing about at the last minute to get everything done you will have to consider all of them at the planning stage. James needs to think about preparing himself for seminars by consolidating notes from lectures and reading, as well as producing the essays. If he is going to achieve this he needs to allocate time each week for his ongoing reading and consolidation, as well as time for the essays. Writing the essay will be the final stage of production. Before he can start this he will need to research the subjects and produce an essay plan; both these activities could form separate learning objectives.

James could also divide the time he spends on essays into preparation and writing time. Four out of the 6 weeks available to him could be spent on preparation and the remaining 2 weeks could be used for writing.

Some people feel that they work well when they are put under pressure. They believe that they are most productive when they are up against a tight deadline. There is nothing wrong with this approach if you are sure that you have the skills to carry it off. However, there are some disadvantages that go along with it, which you may like to consider before you decide it is your preferred option.

Think about:

- *The availability of resources. If you leave everything until the last minute you can succeed only if everything you need is in the right place at the right time. If you need to borrow books from the library or you require access to computers you will be competing with all the other people who have put themselves (by accident or design) in the same position. There is more on this in Chapter 4, which looks at using information technology.*

- *The research that you need to complete before you can start writing. The adrenaline that starts to flow if you leave things until the last minute may help you to write faster but you will not be able to produce good-quality work unless you develop a thorough knowledge of the material. Before you commit yourself to paper you will need to get to grips with the theories and concepts you are writing about. You will need to know what other people have written or said before you can establish you own point of view. Make sure that you allow yourself time for preparation, as well as for writing. There is more on this in Chapter 9, which looks at developing an argument.*

DEFINING PRIORITIES

Effective management of your time will involve defining priorities. If everything is left until the last minute then everything seems to be a priority. If you are aware of long-term and short-term goals this situation can be avoided. If pieces of work have different submission dates then the earliest becomes a potential priority. If you ignore all the other work to complete it in time you may miss the other submission dates. To meet all the dates you need to devote some time to maintaining work that is not an immediate priority. If you devote three-quarters of your study time to completing your first assignment then it would be a good idea to spend the remaining quarter doing some preparatory reading for the assignment that follows. This is evidence of effective long-term planning.

This chapter has talked about the advantages of making schedules and timetables. It is worth remembering that they are there to help you and not to hinder you. If they prevent you from thinking about a situation from a new angle then you may benefit from a different approach. It will not help you if the process becomes oppressive. Try to avoid being ruled and constrained by plans. If an assignment takes much longer than you expected it may make sense to put all of your energy into completing it. Adopting a different approach can be seen as evidence of flexibility and responsiveness. Under some circumstances it may be wise to assess the relevance of long-term goals and introduce some measures to deal with immediate needs and priorities. When you have completed the assignment it may be possible to catch up with your reading through judicious time management (or spending a couple of nights in rather than going out).

Planning and goals are not only important in relation to assignments and essays. They also help you to structure your approach to different subjects. For example, a Diploma in Nursing Studies has 'core' themes, which reflect different academic disciplines. You may be tempted to get hooked into one theme and ignore the others. This can happen if you like one subject more than the others or if you find one subject more difficult than the others.

Developing a special interest in a particular subject, or knowing that a subject is likely to be your Achilles heel, can be beneficial. Having this knowledge shows that you are aware of your strengths and weaknesses. It can become a disadvantage if preferences encourage you to avoid work related to other subjects. Remember that they have the potential to become problems as well. Being aware of how much time you dedicate to each area will help you to avoid getting hooked into a single theme. It may make you more conscious of the need to maintain a consistent approach to your studies. This does not mean that you have to spend equal amounts of time on each. It may involve making thoughtful decisions and keeping records so that you know how you are using your study time.

THINKING STRATEGICALLY

Creating a plan is useful even if you do not stick to it. Departing from your schedule may be beneficial if an unforeseen event becomes a priority. Even if you find that you constantly have to change your plans or reorganize your priorities, it is still a productive way of working. Planning means that you have to think about what you are going to do and why you are going to do it. Planning is evidence of thinking strategically. Developing a strategy for learning is an antidote to drifting aimlessly or bumping along from one crisis to the next. Forward planning and thinking things over before you take decisions gives you some control over future events. It may not enable you to predict everything that is going to happen, but it will make you aware of some of the options at your disposal. This can boost your self-confidence and allow you to take a more positive approach to course work.

Students think about their work in different ways. Some people will visualize plans as a series of tasks arranged in a hierarchical order. The most important task will be at the top of an imaginary list. Strategies may involve devising ways of working down the list until all the tasks are completed. Other people may imagine an hourly timetable with time slots allocated to different subjects and activities. Strategies may involve working out how many hours will be required to complete an essay or how much time is required for background reading prior to a weekly seminar. The following sort of questions may run through your mind:

- Where is there a couple of hours free so that I can visit the library?
- When can I find an hour to read about the composition of the blood? I can make notes to clarify some of the things I did not understand during the lecture.
- I need to make a plan before I can start writing this essay. Where will I find the time to make a start?

Whether you approach an activity by thinking of it as a task or as a period of time is less important than the fact that you are aware of the need to make space for it. Defining the task and creating a space for it are the key ingredients in any plan. The ways in which you mix them together are up to you!

A successful plan will be built around a realistic appraisal of your own habits. You may decide to try and work using long periods for learning rather than more frequent shorter bouts. This can be useful if you want to tackle some big tasks in one go. This approach will not suit everyone. If you know that your concentration span is between 20 and 30 minutes then periods of between 2 and 3 hours will not be the best option. Even if you set this amount of time aside you may only work for 20 minutes in each hour because you become distracted after a short time. This results in a lot of time being wasted. You may end up feeling angry and frustrated. Instead of big chunks you may need to plan so that you have shorter but more frequent periods of study. You may do less in each session but you will stand a better chance of maintaining your interest and enthusiasm if you work in a way that suits you.

There is no single method for drawing up plans that is going to meet every student's needs. Everyone works and studies in the way that suits them. You may like to try some of the suggestions in this chapter to see if they suit you. Don't worry if they do not. Experimentation is a way of finding out what is best for you. Try a variety of methods and see which seems to be the most effective.

Because no one else can prescribe a way of managing your time so that all your needs are met, you will need to evaluate the situation yourself. Making an evaluation of your own progress is one aspect of reflection. Reflection is discussed in more detail in Chapter 11; you may like to glance at this chapter and make some notes on key points, or spend some time reading it when you have completed this section. Ask yourself the following questions so that you think about the effectiveness of your current study habits:

- *Are other activities interfering with my study activities?*
- *Do my goals and priorities suit my current needs?*
- *Am I allowing myself enough time to study?*
- *Is my weekly timetable flexible enough to allow for the unexpected?*
- *Does my weekly schedule show that I am wasting time?*
- *Have I established a good balance between work and leisure in my schedule?*

The answers to these questions may make you change your habits or amend your timetable. It is unlikely that you will get it absolutely right the first time you do it. Adjustments and amendments are ways of adapting you original ideas so that they meet your current requirements.

A PLACE TO STUDY

The ideal is to have your own desk, bookcase and computer in your own room. For most people this ideal is not possible and a place to study is a dining room table or some other shared space. Strains can be put on relationships if others are doing all the accommodating, such as giving you free time by taking on extra domestic chores. Expecting the family to eat their meals on their knees in the lounge because you have commandeered the dining table may be all right for the odd occasion, but will be tolerated for only so long. You are more likely to get continued support if you can minimize the disruption that your need for space can create. In this kind of situation strategies need to be devised to meet everyone's needs.

When you are studying you are likely to have a lot of material around you – writing paper, textbooks and journal articles, lecture

FIGURE 1.2

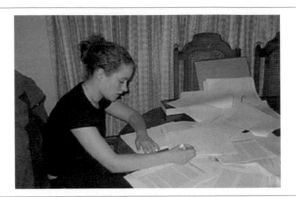

FIGURE 1.3

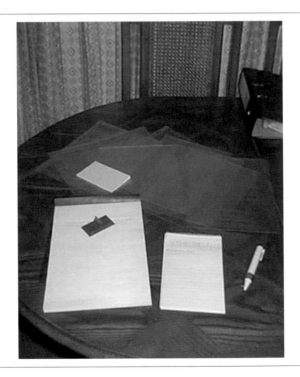

notes and handouts and so on. This can not only clutter your table
but also create a sense of chaos (Fig. 1.2).

By having a few organizational materials to hand you can
make life much easier (Fig. 1.3). Semi-adhesive tabs are useful for
keeping a page, so you can close a book and still go back to the piece

FIGURE 1.4

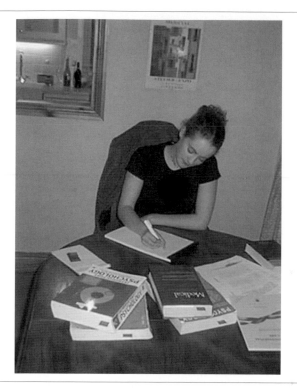

you were referring to. Post-it notes can be used for this purpose, or to jot notes if you don't want to write in the margin of books. Sometimes stray thoughts can pop into your mind and disrupt the creative flow – deal with these by jotting them down on a note pad, so you know they won't be forgotten, then get back to the work in hand.

Figure 1.4 shows what a difference this approach can make to your workspace.

Try to develop good organizational habits, such as only having the material you need at hand. It is tempting, after a long study session, just to leave them there; after all, you know where everything is and you can simply sit down and start work again when you are ready. But this may not be what your flatmates, children or partner want, so think of their needs. One fairly cheap but effective way of keeping everyone happy, including yourself, is to buy a box-file and a few clear plastic wallets for your current project. Your own work-to-date can go in one wallet, lecture notes and handouts can go in another and any photocopied papers can be stored in another. These will all be kept

FIGURE 1.5

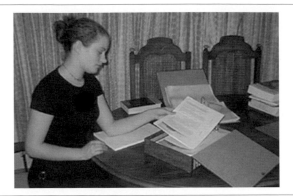

in the box file without any danger of becoming strewn all over the place or accidentally separated (Fig. 1.5). It can be very frustrating if someone has used the nearest piece of paper to hand to write a telephone message or shopping list, when that paper happens to be your draft essay, which you will never be able to reproduce in exactly the way you had written it!

Using study periods

Having considered time and place arrangements you now need to think how you will use your study time effectively.

Think back to previous courses, or times when you have had to study hard:
- *How easy was it to just sit down and start?*
- *How long did you spend on each separate topic?*
- *How often did you take breaks? – for how long? – what did you do?*
- *How did you manage your tension?*

There is a great deal of difference between spending a lot of time feeling very anxious amongst your books and studying effectively, so you will need to consider each of these points.

Creating a suitable environment

When you have determined when and what you are going to study you will need to decide where you are going to do it. Some activities require a specialized environment like a library or access to computers.

BOX 1.1

Getting started – students often say that this is one of the most difficult things to do. The range of avoidance strategies they give is fascinating; first, every pencil they own has to be sharpened, then a cup of tea or coffee is essential, and then perhaps a look at the crossword to 'get the brain in gear'. Some have even ironed shirts or made biscuits because it is simply not possible to do any study until you have done 'something useful'!

In a word, this is procrastination. It is as if studying is a foreign process and these activities are the body's natural response to it. Be sensible, you can live without home-made biscuits, honestly!

The length of your sessions – try to break up your study time into 30–40-minute periods and take short breaks in between. Now you can sharpen pencils or even iron a few clothes (but not many, and you definitely can't make biscuits!). You will be surprised how refreshed you feel after turning your mind to something trivial for a few minutes. It seems a shame that having conquered your fear of starting to study you should even consider stopping. However, long, unbroken study sessions are inefficient because they lead to fatigue; the longer you carry on, the less effective you are likely to be. If you are revising, or learning new material, you will remember less of the later material than that which you read earlier. If you are writing an essay you will find ideas harder to develop and express the longer you go on.

Managing tension – be aware of your body. Intense mental activity can generate tension, which may act as a barrier to learning. If you find your muscles tightening and your fists clenching then you need to relax; these are symptoms of adrenaline (epinephrine) release, which occurs when the body is under stress. Adrenaline prepares the body to deal with the causes of stress, and creates the 'fight or flight' syndrome, but you have nothing to fight and nothing to flee from – you are only reading and writing. Perhaps you need to 'burn off' this adrenaline; as your body is prepared for physical action then do something physical, like going for a jog (or a brisk walk for the less energetic) – perhaps a little light gardening or back to the ironing board with a vengeance. Ten minutes or so is not such a loss from your study time if it helps prepare you for another session with the books.

Muscular tension may also be caused by poor posture, for example being hunched over books or a computer keyboard. This may lead to tension headaches or a general feeling of fatigue. If you notice these symptoms then make a conscious effort to adjust your posture.

On these occasions you will need to plan ahead so that you are in the right place at the right time. On other occasions you will be able to exercise more choice and select where you work. Some people prefer to work in the spaces provided by the university, such as workstations in a library or reading room. These places are set aside for studying so they are free from distractions. Other people like to work at home with familiar things around them. If you prefer this option you may like to think about putting some space aside for studying on a regular basis. This is part of encouraging 'regular' study habits; it may amount to nothing more than somewhere to leave your books and notes out where they are not disturbed and it may mean making some adjustments so that your existing space or room provides you with a more conducive environment.

- Make sure there is adequate light, heating and ventilation – you will not be able to work effectively if it is stuffy in the summer or freezing in the winter
- Try and get a table or desk that is large enough to take all your books, papers, desk lamp, etc.
- Find a place close at hand to store dictionaries, files with notes and textbooks
- Try and use a room where you can be on your own for a while so that you can avoid distractions
- Choose a chair that will enable you to sit and read without causing you any discomfort.

DEVELOPING NETWORKS FOR SUPPORT

The material that you have read earlier in this chapter indicates that studying can become a big thing in your life. It can impinge on your social life, your family and your relationships with partners and friends. If you are moving to another city to start a degree or diploma then the changes in your life may be accompanied by the entire trauma that goes along with moving your possessions, bank, etc. You may also be leaving home, your parents or your partner. You may look forward to the challenge or you may be anxious because you will have to make sense of all these changes on your own in an unfamiliar place. One way of reducing your anxiety is to talk to people you know about the way you feel. They may not be able to make the unpleasant feelings go away but they can provide reassurance.

- *What can be gained from moving to a new place? What does the accommodation, town or city you are moving to have to offer?*
- *What can you gain from starting a new course? Will you have an opportunity to meet new friends or colleagues? Will you have a chance to talk about things that interest you or things that you are concerned about?*

If you are staying at home, studying may be just as traumatic. Spending time at university or immersing yourself in course work means there is less time to do the things you already do. This includes things like the housework and gardening, as well as time spent with children or partners. Creating time and space to study can involve negotiating with the people around you. If you need peace and quiet to get things done then you need to let other people know where and when you are going to study. If you are going to invest a lot of time in your studies you need to sort out who is going to do the jobs that you will not have time for. Students with course work, homes and children will have to enter into negotiations with their families so that they can share or delegate domestic work and childcare. You may have to discuss your changing responsibilities and how studying will change your role. When you are allocated to placements you will often also be allocated a mentor or supervisor. You may find that you have similar discussions with them regarding your role in the area and your responsibilities as a learner. In both cases negotiation will be necessary to establish: what you expect, and what is expected from you; what you intend to do, and what other people think you should do; and how you are going to organize yourself and other people so that it all gets done. There is further discussion about mentors and supervisors in Chapter 2.

CASE STUDY

Joan has recently started a post-registration course. Her employers have agreed to give her study time so that she can attend the parts of the course that are taught at the university. She also knows that she will need more time to complete the project work and essays that are specified in the course requirements.

Joan has two children at school and she is worried about the commitments that she already has. These include managing her responsibilities at work, her work at home and childcare, Mike, her partner, has encouraged her to take the course and gain more qualifications but he has not said how he is going to support her while she is studying. Mike has done the housework and looked after the children when Joan has made a specific request for help but he has never used his initiative and done things without a request from her.

Put yourself in Joan's shoes.
- Where should Joan go for help and advice?
- How should she sort things out with Mike?

If you are finding things difficult it may be helpful to talk to other people who are in a similar situation. Remember that some of the people you meet on the first day of the course are going to be in the same position as you. They may have ways of coping that you have not thought of. Even if they do not have solutions to your problems, they may be able to sympathize with you, which can be a source of comfort. If there are other people who share your problems and concerns it may be possible to form a self-help group, which will encourage group members to provide support and advice for each other.

Another strategy is to see what the university can offer. Some courses may allocate you a personal tutor who will be able to offer advice on personal problems as well as problems related to course work. Some student unions have health and welfare officers who can advise on problems related to accommodation or access to resources. You may also have access to a counsellor if you do not want to approach any of the people mentioned above.

- Look for references to any of these people in your university handbook
- Look for references to them in any material that you receive from the National Union of Students (NUS)
- Look for information on notice boards
- Make a note if they are mentioned in any presentations made by the staff during your introduction to the university
- Listen to other students; they may recommend someone who has worked with them to overcome a problem
- See if there are any clubs or societies that you want to join. They are a good way of making friends and meeting people who share common interests

It is always worthwhile attending orientation sessions and picking up handbooks. You may not need to contact any of these people straight away but it is useful to know who and where they are in case you require their services in the future.

During this chapter you have considered timetabling and organization. Remember the following key points when you begin to study:

- Acknowledge your other commitments
- Make realistic plans
- Think strategically
- Create a structure by setting aims and objectives, goals, or more urgent and less urgent priorities
- Evaluate and reflect on your learning
- Be prepared to seek and accept help and advice from other people

CHAPTER RESOURCES

REFERENCE

Northedge A 1990 The good study guide. Open University, Milton Keynes

2 Learning skills and learning styles

Ian Welsh with Sian Maslin-Prothero

KEY ISSUES

- **What learning is**
- **Understanding memory**
- **Responsibility for your own learning**
- **Learning styles**
- **Your existing learning skills**
- **Learning from life experiences**
- **Learning contracts**
- **Support networks**
- **Self-assessment**

INTRODUCTION

Chapter 1 was about managing your resources so that you can study effectively. The overall aim of this chapter is to build on the previous one and develop your learning skills. This will be achieved by identifying what learning is and how we do it. There will be an explanation of different learning styles and how they can affect your studying and an opportunity to identify your personal learning style. Knowing how you prefer to learn can help guide you through your course, although you need to be aware that your preference can change according to what you are studying.

WHAT IS LEARNING?

Learning is something we do practically every day so it may seem a bit strange to be asking what we mean by it. However, knowing how learning occurs may help you to become a more effective learner. This section is about the process of learning and what goes on while we are doing it.

Learning can be defined as *any more or less permanent change in behaviour, knowledge or belief*. In order to experience the change we need to be exposed to new ideas or skills. Sometimes we are not conscious of the exposure as a learning experience – if you can recite an advertising slogan or sing a jingle (quietly, you don't want to draw attention to yourself!) you will have proved that you can learn without trying. This is known as passive learning, which is due to frequent

FIGURE 2.1   *The progression from acquisition of knowledge to active learning*

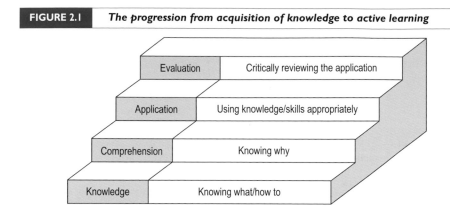

exposure. You can learn more useful things this way, for example the signs and symptoms of diseases you frequently encounter in clinical practice. Such learning, however, is superficial because you may not necessarily understand why they occur. Likewise, you can copy the skills you have observed a more experienced practitioner perform, but will you be able to modify the skill when a new and slightly different situation occurs?

Passive learning is an inevitable feature of life but professional practice is more than just copying the behaviour of our predecessors and learning facts by rote. The Code of Professional Conduct requires practitioners to 'maintain your professional knowledge and competence' (Nursing and Midwifery Council 2002, para. 6). This means that you must actively engage in the learning process. Active learning occurs when the student sets out to understand the principles behind the concepts and skills they are studying. It may help to view learning as a progression from the acquisition of knowledge through to higher level mental activities (Fig. 2.1).

Figure 2.1 represents the progression starting from being able to remember straightforward facts, such as being able to label a diagram of the heart (simple recall or knowing what the various parts are). This is a useful starting point but it constitutes only a part of learning.

Being able to explain the function of the heart valves, or the reason why the muscle layer of the left ventricle is thicker than the right represents a higher level of learning – the ability to comprehend the concepts you are studying.

Going beyond this level is the stage of being able to put your knowledge to use (application). For example, if you have a patient who has suffered damage to the left ventricle following a coronary thrombosis you will be able to plan nursing care that takes the patient's impaired circulation into account.

By observing the effect of exercise on the patient, such as the degree of breathlessness after walking a prescribed distance, you will be able to evaluate the effect your plan has had on the patient's heart.

Simply knowing and being able to perform are important but lower order activities. This is the level of the worker who just has to follow orders. Students such as yourself are studying to be able to act independently and to exercise professional judgement, therefore passive learning is not enough; active participation in the learning process is essential.

So learning is more than the mere acquisition of facts, it involves a range of intellectual activities including the ability to make judgements on abstract matters such as topical issues or ethics.

Think about some of your political, religious or ethical beliefs.

- How did you acquire them?
- Do you understand the principles upon which they are based?
- How do they affect your practice?
- Have you at any time subjected them to serious critical scrutiny?

Quite often our beliefs are picked up from influential people around us, such as parents, religious ministers or teachers, and we accept them because we respect the authority of the person who is teaching us; we expect them to know what they are talking about. Such learning may be passive, due to being constantly exposed to the same ideas since childhood. Even discussions with friends or family with the same views may not encourage a critical perspective.

SO HOW DO WE LEARN?

The concepts of learning and memory are closely related. When we need to perform a skill, recall an item of knowledge or explain something, we draw on our memory. But we can only pull out what is already there. Knowing how memory works may help you develop effective learning skills. Although memory is an incompletely understood concept, one theory may have some practical use. The Atkinson–Schiffrin model, described by Malim and Birch (1998, p. 291) explains memory as a series of steps (Fig. 2.2).

We are bombarded every second with sensory inputs – stop for a moment and try to focus on the information that you are receiving now via your five senses. This tells you what is happening outside your body; so also focus on what your body is telling you about inside you – have you any discomfort, aches and pains, is your bladder full?! Without looking, are your knees straight or flexed?

| FIGURE 2.2 | *The Atkinson–Schiffrin model of memory* (adapted from Malim and Birch 1998, reproduced with permission of Palgrave) |

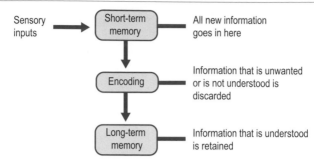

All of this information is coming at you while you are trying to learn from a lecture or demonstration and all of it goes into your short-term memory. That is to say, every second you are gaining a mass of information, most of which you don't need. For example, sensations you experience during a lecture, traffic noise, the smell of fresh paint, have no relevance. All sensory inputs are encoded – we try to give them meaning – those that have no relevance now are discarded. If you can understand lecture material, i.e. it makes sense to you, you can give it meaning in relation to your own experience then you have successfully encoded it and it will enter and remain in your long-term memory. If you can't make sense of it, it will not be retained. Only information stored in the long-term memory can be recalled.

Memory, therefore, is very much dependent on learning – making sense of information.

- Try to recall the definition of learning
- Describe the difference between active and passive learning
- What effect can distractions, such as music or television have on the encoding part of memory?

To make sense of new material (the encoding process), we have to work hard to establish links between what we already know and the new information. Consider the following example.

When studying orthopaedics you come across the term *subperiosteal cellular proliferation*. At first glance you may just see a complicated medical term, but when you look carefully you will see that there are some familiar components:

Sub – means below
Peri – means around

Cellular – refers to cells
Proliferation – production of a large number.

So you can work out that a large number of cells are being produced, but where exactly? You have to try to understand the meaning of *subperiosteal*. At this point you may need a medical dictionary to look up the meaning of *periosteal* (around the bone – *os* is Latin for bone). Looking at a diagram of a bone in an anatomy book will show you that the periosteum is the tissue that surrounds bone, so *subperiosteal* refers to the site below the periosteum where the cells are produced, hence *cellular proliferation*.

Making sense of something like this is an encoding process – you are making sense of it.

As you will know from your own experience, making new links does not always happen the first time you try to learn something. Constant effort is required. If you can recall a time when you learned a skill, such as how to play tennis, to dance, or even to play a board game like chess, you will remember how you got some things right and some things wrong. Eventually, as you persevered you became relatively skilful and were able to perform in a fairly fluent way. It is believed that when we are learning we are making new circuits between our neurons (brain cells). These neural pathways are physical structures and are activated when we need to recall something. It may be helpful to use an analogy to explain this concept.

Think about a number of towns without any road or rail links; communication between them would be impossible. Laying down new roads and railway lines is a difficult and time-consuming job but, once they have been established, traffic can travel rapidly between the towns.

And so it is with learning, once the hard work of understanding new concepts and developing new skills has been done, the neural pathways have been established and the information traffic can speed rapidly around the brain. This is why learning has been described as a more or less permanent change.

So why do we forget?

Perhaps the question should be 'have we really learned?' Spending time and effort does not necessarily guarantee success in learning, it is how we use it that is important. Figure 2.3 shows the effect when the student is stimulated to recall information, or practice skills, soon after being exposed to them and if they do this frequently, the chances

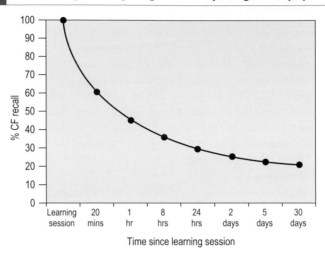

FIGURE 2.3   *The Ebbinghaus Forgetting Curve – improving memory by recall*

of forgetting are reduced. The frequency of recall is the key factor in remembering.

The main principle is to give yourself as many opportunities as possible to rehearse. If this means practising a skill then do so as often as you can and as soon as possible after being taught. For knowledge and understanding try to set yourself a series of short tests, based on the information you have read or been taught.

The memories of concepts that we have learned and skills that we can perform are stored in the long-term memory and are recalled when we need them.

Sometimes, though, perhaps because of anxiety, we fail to recall them, such as during an examination. You may have had the experience of not being able to answer a question in an exam and then, when you leave the room, the answer comes to you in a flash. One way of dealing with this is to visualize the brain as a channel that is constricted, preventing the flow of information. Relaxation techniques may be helpful in situations like this. By imagining the relaxation of the walls of the channel you can imagine the flow returning.

You may feel that you do not have time to close your eyes and relax your body during an exam situation but if the alternative is not answering a question do you have anything to lose? You may find that by relaxing and thinking loosely about the question some ideas may begin to spark off and that these lead to other relevant ideas. In other words, the information traffic starts to flow again.

KNOWING THINGS

How can we know anything? For example, how do you know that the South Pole exists? Or how do you know that oxygen moves into cells? The chances are that you 'know' because someone told you. This type of knowledge is second-hand knowledge – sometimes known as propositional knowledge.

Is there a difference between knowing and knowing about? You may know about the native inhabitants of Australia but how deep is your knowledge? Do you know them as well as someone who has lived with them?

WHERE DOES KNOWLEDGE COME FROM?

The second-hand knowledge that has been passed on to you had to originate somewhere. All the science, history, bits of geography and information that you have acquired started as someone's experience. Knowledge can be described as the articulation of human experience. Once someone has experienced something, such as discovering oxygen or the quickest route from one place to another, it can be described, i.e. articulated, or made known to others. In order to gain knowledge that is more than second-hand you need to have a significant experience from which to learn.

Kolb, an influential thinker on experiential learning, stated that 'Learning is the process whereby knowledge is created through the transformation of experience' (Kolb 1984). He was referring to the development of personal, as opposed to propositional knowledge; that is to say you know rather than merely know about something.

BEING AN ADULT LEARNER

One of the points that will be emphasized on any course of study is the importance of taking responsibility for your own learning. Higher education is very different from school. At school, it was your teachers who were responsible for identifying what and how you learned. As an adult learner, it is up to you to identify what you want to learn and how much effort you are going to give to learning. That is, only you can successfully complete this course.

This book aims to help you in becoming an independent and self-directed learner. This means you will be able to identify what you need to learn and access the information you require without the assistance of a teacher. There will be additional mechanisms in your place of learning to support and assist you during the course, but you need to recognize how you take responsibility for your own learning.

Perhaps the first thing to realize is that when you enter a professional course in a university or college you have earned the right to be there; you have passed a rigorous selection procedure. The reason I make this point is that quite often adult students carry negative perceptions of themselves if they feel that they 'could have done better at school'. There may also be a sense of inferiority in relation to the lecturers. This stems from the power relationships that existed between you as a child and your teachers as adults in authority. As an adult learner you enter education with the status of an adult, a range of experiences and the motivation to gain a qualification. You are there because you choose to be – this is not compulsory education. Psychologists call this 'intrinsic motivation', the strongest driving force there is.

A key proponent to any success is motivation – a sense of purpose is perhaps the most crucial aspect of learning. You must want to study. For example, if you are undertaking a pre-registration nursing course because you couldn't think of anything else to do, you are not increasing your chances of success. The driving force, or motivation, is weak.

The reason why motivation is so important when you are embarking on something new and challenging, such as a course, is that there are going to be times when you find the going difficult. You will find that, regardless of what you have identified as motivating you at the start of a new course, your motivation changes during the course.

Briefly note down what has motivated you, either to start a new course or to learn a new skill.

Sometimes your motivation is going to be better, sometimes worse. This might be for a variety of reasons. You might have concerns about:

- financial insecurity
- meeting new people
- having reduced time available for family and friends
- making time for study
- not understanding the course and/or the academic language used by your teachers and peers.

A new course is exciting; however, it is going to bring about a change in your life. This change might cause you stress. Stress is not always a negative thing; only when you are experiencing too much pressure does it become a problem. An adequate amount of pressure stimulates us and can be a very positive thing. However, if not managed correctly, this pressure can become too much and we are unable to cope, leading to too much pressure. It is important to be able to recognize these signs and symptoms in yourself and others. Only through recognition and then doing something to create a change will you adequately address the problem. Chapter 1 identified some positive strategies that can be used to resolve some of these issues.

LEARNING STYLES

Learning underpins everything we do, for example learning to drive, trying out a new recipe or learning to rock climb. We rarely stop and think how we have learned a new skill. During the course your teachers will support your learning through a variety of teaching and learning strategies including lectures, seminars, tutorials and practice.

Too often both students and teachers believe that the teacher is the 'expert' and knower of all things. First of all, this is untrue: we are all constantly learning new things and developing new skills. Becoming dependent on teachers will stifle your creativity and your ability to make independent judgements and utilize new information. As identified previously, you will find that your teachers will expect you to take responsibility for your own learning, through making the most of every opportunity offered you.

What you will find is that we all learn in different ways. This will be based on your previous experiences, and how you have learned to learn in the past. To be successful you need to identify how you learn best and develop your learning style so that you can optimize any learning situation as it presents itself.

Honey and Mumford (1992) identified four basic learning styles: the activist, the reflector, the pragmatist and the theorist. Box 2.1 summarizes each of these different styles.

BOX 2.1	*Learning styles*

The Activist

- Enjoys new experiences and challenges
- Enjoys an environment of changing activities
- Likes being the centre of attention
- Appreciates the chance to develop ideas through interaction and discussion with others.

The activist will thrive and develop in an environment that utilizes some of the following teaching and learning strategies: group work, seminars, discussions, debates and workshops.

The Reflector

■ Appreciates the opportunity to reflect prior to making a decision or choice

■ Prefers to listen and observe others debating and discussing issues

■ Would choose to work independently of others.

The reflector is someone who prefers to work on their own, through individual study and project work. They are likely to prefer lectures.

The Pragmatist

■ Likes linking theory with practice

■ Enjoys problem-solving

■ Appreciates the opportunity to develop practical skills.

The pragmatist will enjoy those learning experiences that involve problem-solving activities, practical sessions, clinical experiences and work-based projects.

The Theorist

■ Enjoys theories and models

■ Thrives on problem-solving, which involves understanding and making sense of complex issues

■ Likes structure and making the link to theories.

The theorist will benefit and enjoy those sessions that use problem-solving, evaluating material and discussing theories with colleagues and teachers.

You have probably identified your preferred learning style from what has been listed, and this will help guide you and recognize those situations from which you might learn more effectively. You will benefit from developing new skills, which may help you to learn effectively from every situation you encounter. The following are suggestions on how you might develop a new learning style.

BOX 2.2	*Developing your learning styles*

Developing an activist style

■ Diversify. Learn to divide-up your time between activities. For example, read an article, then prepare for tomorrow's lecture, etc.

■ Contribute in discussions and debates. Let people know what you think. Group participation will help you develop your arguments (excellent practice for essay writing). It will also increase your confidence and self-esteem.

Developing a reflector style

■ Spend time thinking things through. Develop plans for assignments.

■ Read around subjects being studied. Think and plan carefully what you are going to write. Discuss these plans with your teacher and fellow students.

■ In discussions, observe what is going on. What are other people saying? How do they react to others in the group?

Developing a pragmatist style

■ Have a go at linking the theory to practice. For example, do a literature review using the CD-ROM, have a go at practising your basic life-support skills on a mannikin.

■ Ask others to observe what you are practising and to give constructive feedback; assess yourself too.

Developing a theorist style

■ Develop your analytical skills. Compare and contrast two conflicting ideas.

■ Discuss your findings with colleagues. What did they find?

Record your learning preferences in your reflective diary (see page 38). Note down if your preference changes. Are these changes according to what subject is being learned?

You will find that your preferred learning style might change depending on your needs or who is facilitating the session. The important thing is to learn to be flexible and to develop your skills.

LEARNING FROM LIFE EXPERIENCES

In many vocational courses, such as nursing or midwifery, there is criticism of the so called 'theory–practice gap' (Rolfe 1996). Practitioners often say that what is taught in the classroom is quite different from what is practised on the wards. In fact, what is taught within the university or college is a theoretical underpinning of practice. Practice itself, for the most part, is taught in the wards, departments and community by practitioners; that is why the courses are usually equally divided between university or college and clinical placements.

However, this is not to say that clinical placements only provide opportunity for practice; it is my contention that a substantial amount of theoretical learning can be acquired through practice if certain conditions are met. This section will deal with:

■ learning through experience
■ student–mentor relationships
■ using clinical assessments as learning experiences
■ integration of theory with practice.

All of these relate to your forthcoming clinical learning opportunities.

| FIGURE 2.4 | *Kolb's experiential learning cycle* |

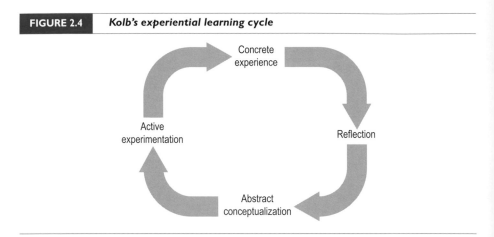

Does having an experience necessarily result in learning?

In Kolb's view, experiential learning is a process that results in the generation of new knowledge, insights, ideas and even new skills. He described the process as an *experiential learning cycle* (Fig. 2.4).

A *concrete experience* is an event that happens to an individual, which, in the context of learning, provides the learning focus, for example, learning to play a musical instrument or learning to give an injection.

Reflection is the process of thinking about the experience in a structured way. Schon (1983) stated that reflection on action is 'a retrospective view of an experience to uncover the knowledge used in a particular situation'. Neither Schon nor Kolb describe in detail how an individual could reflect. Other writers, such as Gibbs (1988), Johns (1994) and Boud et al (1985) have offered ideas on how the reflective process can be structured (see Chapter 11). The model of reflection developed by Boud et al (1985) is relatively simple but also academically rigorous. Boud et al recommend that reflection should be on three aspects of the experience:

- **Actions** – what you and any other participants did in the situation you are reflecting on
- **Feelings** – your negative and/or positive feelings, and the reasons why you felt the way you did
- **Knowledge** – the existing knowledge you had that was of use at the time, and the knowledge you realized you lack.

Reflection is not simply a matter of remembering an event and thinking 'that was interesting/unpleasant/embarrassing' or whatever, it is a structured process designed to enhance your own understanding and develop fresh insights.

Nursing is a practical job – so why is it important to spend time reflecting on it?

Abstract conceptualization follows on from reflection. A concept is an idea; abstract conceptualization is your understanding of a concept. For example, you may have some understanding of the way blood pressure is maintained and how it changes during different physical activities. When we reflect in a systematic way we gain new insights and develop knowledge and understandings that we did not have previously. This may be in the form of theoretical knowledge, such as learning about the pressure receptors in the lining of blood vessels and their role in regulating blood pressure or it might be through gaining insights into your own feelings – why you feel uncomfortable in certain situations, which, once you have some deeper self-awareness, you can act on to make yourself more confident.

Once you have spent time reflecting and reorganizing your personal knowledge and insights you will be ready for active experimentation, ready to have another go at the experience but with fresh ideas. Reflection therefore, is a way of improving your insights into nursing practice and improving the practice itself (see Chapters 11 and 13).

By using a systematic process, such as the one described by Kolb, allied with a structured model of reflection, you will be demonstrating an analytical approach to the practical activity of nursing. This will enhance your understanding of the theoretical principles that underpin nursing practice. Obviously you will not be able to do this for every single activity you engage in, but if you can develop the habit of reflecting on certain events that have some significance for you, you will amass a great amount of useful knowledge to help you nurse patients with understanding, rather than as a matter of performing routines.

Becoming a reflective practitioner

Like any other skill, reflective practice can be learned and, once learned, can become second nature. In order to reflect effectively a number of conditions need to be met.

- You need to **set aside some time.** Reflection is more than allowing the day's events to run through your head on your way home.
- You need **the support of a mentor**, to help direct your thoughts, to pass on their own insights and generally to provide a sympathetic ear.

- You need to create **a framework to structure reflections**, such as the one described by Boud et al (1985).
- You need **a predisposition to reflect**, that is to say, a tendency to take a reflective view of significant life events. Many people have this predisposition but, without the other three factors, they tend not to develop their reflective skills.

Analysis of the scores from a group of nursing students who had completed a 'learning styles' questionnaire showed that the most predominant learning style was the reflective style. Clearly most (but not all) have got the predisposition that will help them derive knowledge from practice. That is to say, they will have the advantage of developing personal knowledge and not merely rely on propositional knowledge. This knowledge is more permanent, useful in practice and invaluable in examinations.

REFLECTIVE DIARIES

As identified earlier, we all learn in different ways. Learning through reflection helps us to focus on the material that interests us. We can learn more quickly if the material is relevant and interesting to us. By drawing on your own personal knowledge and life experience you can try out and test new ideas and concepts. That is learning by doing, practising and occasionally making mistakes. Through feedback from others, such as our mentors (as well as ourselves), absorbing what has been said and making sense of what has been said, we then progress. It is important to see this as a continuous process. We might not think of it consciously but when we stop and think 'How did I get here?' we are able to follow this process.

One way of assisting this process is through a reflective diary. Keeping a reflective diary will enable you to:

- record details as they occur
- remember things that happened
- organize and clarify thoughts
- apply your experiences
- assess your development
- take a longer-term view.

This reflective diary will be your own personal record, to record your thoughts and feelings about colleagues, teachers and clients. You will find it very therapeutic to express your thoughts and feelings and, throughout this book, you will be encouraged to record your experiences in a reflective diary. However, you need to be sure that confidentiality is maintained and that individuals cannot be identified, should anyone else read it.

How to go about developing your reflective diary:

- Set aside 5–10 minutes a day
- Use a framework for reflection, such as the Boud et al (1985) model described above

- Discuss your thoughts and feelings with your clinical mentor

Two examples of student reflections, using this model, are given below. One relates to the care of a stroke patient and the other to an assessment interview. Note how this model has been used in the two entirely different situations.

Lisa's reflection

Using the Boud et al (1985) reflective framework, together with my own reflective diary, I am able to examine in depth my reactions to incidents that have occurred during my training. I can consider how, with a different approach or greater knowledge, I could improve a similar situation if it arose again.

I have recently worked on a ward where many patients had suffered a cerebrovascular accident (CVA), which had resulted in severe communication difficulties. On two occasions on the same shift, different patients attracted my attention and, whilst I dealt with both people immediately, they did not initially appear distressed, so I assumed that their need was not urgent. The first patient, an elderly gentleman, seemed to be motioning towards his table; my first conclusions were that he wanted either his drink or the medication that was waiting to be taken. Neither turned out to be the case, he was actually nodding towards the urine bottles that were stored under the sink opposite his bed. Fortunately, in this instance I discovered the need before any embarrassment was caused; he actually seemed to find the scenario quite amusing.

Sadly this was not the case with the second incident, when an elderly lady had a similar requirement. Both another nurse and myself desperately struggled to identify her needs and it was evident that her urgency and our lack of comprehension were increasingly agitating her. We thought we had identified a desire to stretch her legs but, whilst I turned my back to fetch her walking frame, she became doubly incontinent; this caused considerable embarrassment for everyone in the ward, but most particularly for the patient.

Action

Me – *recognized that patients had a care-related need, tried to guess their requirements.*

Patients – *tried desperately to explain what they wanted; one suffered severe embarrassment.*

Feelings

Positive – *I empathized with the patients, fully appreciating their frustration and embarrassment at the sudden lack of such basic skills, not only the communication aspect but also the need for help with toileting. My first reaction was to escape and get someone else to deal with the situation, but I'm proud that I acted professionally and persevered; at least I discovered the needs of one patient.*

Negative – *embarrassed at the suffering caused to the other patient. Extremely frustrated at the difficulties I encountered in trying to understand them. Annoyed that I didn't consider the elimination need first. I made wrong assumptions based on appearances and did not consider that their condition might have influenced how they were acting.*

Knowledge

Existing knowledge – *I knew the patients had suffered a CVA and that their communication skills were impaired. It was my responsibility to try to identify their needs by questioning.*

Knowledge deficit – *the extent to which a CVA affects communication skills – are both reception and expression skills impaired? When accepting responsibility for looking after such patients I should determine from their notes or the nurse looking after them previously the exact extent of their abilities and comprehension.*

I need to find out how best to deal with patients with communication difficulties, particularly when they do understand me but have difficulty in even responding with a 'Yes' or 'No'. Talking to a speech therapist would give me a greater understanding of the problems and would give me the opportunity to seek guidance over the difficulties in communication. As I have chosen child branch, this problem could arise frequently under different circumstances, such as with younger or handicapped children. I need to develop a strategy to identify needs as quickly as possible, maybe starting with structuring questions to deal with the potentially most embarrassing requirements first. This would probably include the need to become more in tune with patients' non-verbal communication skills.

Learning from this reflection

Improving my knowledge as identified above, and making fewer assumptions will enable me to deal with this situation with more competence in the future, which in turn will save my patients from considerable embarrassment and make their lives in hospital easier.

Gail's reflection

On day two of my clinical placement on a children's orthopaedic ward, I was asked by a staff nurse to complete an admission on a patient. I was immediately presented with an abundance of paperwork and was pointed in the direction of the patient. I informed the staff nurse that I hadn't been involved with an admission before, I then expected her to suggest that I watch her first, but she responded by saying 'Oh, there's nothing to it' and quickly flicked through the forms and questions to be filled in with information from the patient.

Though feeling extremely nervous and unsure, I carried out the admission trying to portray competence in order not to cause any added anxieties for the child or parent.

I found myself asking all questions from the preprinted forms as I was unsure of which applied and which ones didn't. I then took the parents around the ward showing them different rooms, e.g. parents room, toilets.

Action

Nurse – asked me to perform a task that she was aware I hadn't implemented or observed previously.

Me – muddled through the procedure not fully understanding what was required.

Patient and parents – looking bemused at some of the questions I asked.

Feelings

Positive – felt satisfaction that I had managed to stay calm and collected, which enabled the procedure to run smoothly. Felt pleased that I had enabled the family to become familiar with their new environment and had given them a warm welcome.

Negative – I felt confused as I was unable to judge whether I had handled the situation competently because I had nothing to compare. Boyd and Fales (1983) relate this feeling of uncertainty to 'inner discomfort', which is the beginning of a reflective episode.

Felt annoyed with the staff nurse because she had an unfair expectation that I was capable of the admission without any prior training or observance of the procedure.

I felt anxious because she offered very little support and showed no awareness of how I must be feeling.

I felt annoyed about imposing inappropriate questions from the forms because I didn't have the knowledge to judge which information was required or not required. I felt anger towards the nurse having placed me in this position. I also felt annoyed with myself for not being more assertive initially where I could have requested to observe first.

Knowledge

Existing knowledge – *I have good communication skills with children and parents from a previous career and as a 'mum'. I am familiar with the layout of the ward.*

Knowledge deficit – *I need to organize opportunities to observe other nurses performing the admission procedure in order to provide me with a measuring tool, and to see the different approaches of asking questions and acquiring information. According to Boyd and Fales (1983) this phase of the reflection process is 'an openness to new information from internal and external sources, with the ability to observe and take in from a variety of perspectives'. I would also benefit from being observed by my mentor in order to gain feedback on my performance.*

I need to acquire a set of admission forms to enable myself to become familiar with the different types of information needed.

I also need to address my need to increase my assertiveness by seeking clarification and asking for support when I need it and not to feel intimidated by particular staff nurses.

In each case you will see that the students have spent time thinking about their experiences. They have used a systematic framework to help structure their thoughts. Although it is not evident from their writings, they also had guidance from a mentor. They also knew, from doing the Honey and Mumford Learning Styles Inventory that they had a strong predisposition to reflect on their practice.

LEARNING CONTRACTS

A learning contract is an agreement between two or more people. We are making informal contracts with people all the time, for example 'If I look after the children while you go for your tutorial today, can I go climbing later in the week?' A learning contract is used when there is an exchange of something, and this can be skills or knowledge. In this context a learning contract is a more formal, written agreement between a lecturer and a student, or a group of students.

Learning contracts (Fig. 2.5) are being used more frequently in education institutions. The philosophy goes hand-in-hand with students taking more responsibility for their own learning. Once you embark on any course you enter into a variety of informal, unwritten agreements, such as attending the course and completing the required number of assignments.

Learning contracts are particularly useful when you have specific learning outcomes or need to negotiate how you are assessed. It can also be used when you want accreditation for prior learning (APL) or accreditation for prior experiential learning (APEL).

FIGURE 2.5 **Example of a learning contract**

Name of student: Su Lin

Name of tutor/practice supervisor: Liam Bryant

Individual learning objective(s)

1) To develop my team working skills both clinically and when

   in university

Plan of action

* Identify at least four skills I need to develop to make me a more

   effective team member

* Undertake an analysis (with a colleague) of my present

   strengths and weaknesses when working in a team

Resources for help

* Revisit notes on teamwork

* A colleague (either from the department or practice area)

   who will help with the analysis

Evidence to show achievement of objectives

* Self-assessment

* Willingness to participate in a team

* Constructive contribution to the team

* Commitments of the team achieved

Date of contract 25.4.2005 **Date to be completed by** 25.5.2005

Signature of student

Signature of tutor/practice supervisor

Learning contracts enable the student to identify, plan, manage and evaluate their own learning. The learner and their supervisor discuss, agree and record what the student wants to achieve and how it is going to be achieved. Both parties then sign the document.

Learning contracts have a number of benefits:

- Everyone is clear about what the goals are and how they will be achieved
- Everyone knows what is expected of them
- Negotiating your contract not only recognizes your needs but also enables you to take responsibility for your learning
- Learning contracts can recognize prior learning, for example APEL, APL.

Learning contracts are useful for both the learner and the supervisor, and enhance their commitment to the learning experience. This form of contract can be used in conjunction with a placement or workplace experience, where more than two people are contributing to the process.

You need to consider a number of points prior to agreeing your contract.

- *What do you want to get out of this experience (your objectives)?*
- *What skills and knowledge will you gain?*
- *How will you reach/achieve your objectives?*
- *What are the deadlines?*
- *How will you demonstrate that you have achieved your objectives?*

It is important to see the learning contract as something important to you, a way of you achieving your goals, with help and support from your supervisor.

Some of you might have experienced undertaking an individual performance review (IPR). This is a form of appraisal that is frequently used in the NHS. This is a form of learning contract and it is a way that you can ensure that things that are important to you, as well as to the organization, are met.

SUPPORT NETWORKS

Chapter 1 referred to your expectations and fears when embarking on a course of study, and emphasized the importance of managing

FIGURE 2.6   *Example of a support network*

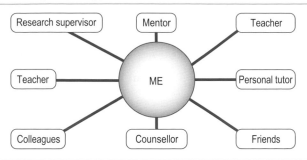

your time. This leads to a more balanced life where you are able to include socializing and successfully studying.

Having identified your preferred learning style, I want to move on and recognize how to get the most out of your supervisors. Supervisors come in a variety of shapes and forms, they can be your teacher, personal tutor, mentor, friend, colleague or research supervisor. A supervisor is an experienced individual who facilitates the development of a colleague both educationally and professionally.

Your supervisor is there to help you learn. This can be in a variety of ways, including: getting the most out of your practice placement, acting as role model, a resource, a counsellor or as a teacher (Fig. 2.6).

The following are key characteristics of a supervisor:

- a good listener
- constructive
- a resource
- a role model
- competent.

However, supervision is not a one-way relationship: your supervisor will have certain expectations of you as a student. Please also remember:

- that supervisors are not only responsible for you, they are usually busy and will have other commitments
- to make appointments to meet your supervisor, and turn up prepared and on time
- to phone if you are unable to make an appointment and let them know you won't be attending.

The emphasis is on you being prepared to listen to the constructive feedback and act on recommendations made. This will require both commitment and work from you. Be prepared to assess yourself and your progress; your learning diary will help you do this. As mentioned previously, supervisors are not gods; they are there to guide your learning, so be prepared and focused in tutorials.

Most practice placements will ensure that you have a mentorship scheme (see Chapter 14). The mentor/supervisor is an experienced nurse, who is there to help make the clinical experience a positive one for you. As with teaching supervisors, you need to establish your relationship, identifying your expectations for the practice placement. Your mentor is responsible for knowing what stage you are at in your course and for helping you to get the most out of your placement experience. It is important that you get to work with your mentor as much as possible. The things that apply with your tutor apply now: organize regular meetings and come to them on time and prepared. Additional points that you need to consider with your mentor include identifying your learning needs while on this placement, whether there is any assessment and when this might be occurring. You will be responsible for any assessment documentation, so look after it and don't leave it lying around (otherwise other people will read it).

What to do when it goes wrong

It is still the case that the majority of students are allocated to a mentor, rather than being able to choose their mentor. Sometimes the relationship does not work. This can be for a variety of reasons, including: not liking each other; your supervisor is unavailable; your requirements have changed. The most important thing is to do something about this. First, you should talk to your mentor and discuss how you are feeling. This might be embarrassing but it will be constructive and allow you to carry on learning.

If it is not possible to resolve any difficulties between you and your supervisor, then you need to identify a replacement mentor.

Study networks

Another way of improving your learning is to form study networks with other students. Study groups are a form of self-help group, and can provide additional support to that which is provided by your teachers. With your fellow students you can:

- share resources
- pool ideas
- brainstorm
- meet and make more friends

- share tasks
- develop group working skills.

You might find you have to initiate the development of a study group. If you are unsure how to do this, approach your teacher for assistance. The following points might help you to develop a study network.

- Organize a meeting
- Explain the purpose of the group
- Decide when, where and how often you will meet
- Keep in touch, exchange addresses and phone numbers
- Meet regularly

ASSESSING YOURSELF

Throughout your career in nursing there is an expectation that you can assess yourself, including your:

- personal skills and qualities
- strengths and weaknesses
- learning requirements.

You will also be expected to learn to evaluate your own work, as well as to evaluate that of others. The ability to assess yourself accurately will be useful in your professional career, as well as a valuable skill from a personal viewpoint. Self-assessment fits well with writing a learning diary. It will help you recognize your learning needs and identify how to achieve them. You will also be able to use it to support feedback received from supervisors, teachers and colleagues.

CONCLUSION

In this chapter you have looked at a variety of essential points necessary to help you with your learning. By identifying your preferred style of learning you can use this information to enhance your studying. In addition, there are costs to learning, and these are not only financial. Support networks are available to make your experience less painful. Finally, the use of learning contracts with supervisors can help you make the most of your learning, and to ensure that you remain in control and that you pace yourself through the course.

Before moving on, take some time and record the following in your reflective diary.

- *What is your preferred learning style?*
- *How will you use this preferred learning style to your advantage?*
- *List the requirements of your ideal supervisor. What do you think they might expect from you?*
- *Identify a supportive friend, with whom you could develop a study network.*
- *Talk to your teacher about learning contracts and developing a learning contract to meet your specific learning needs.*

CHAPTER RESOURCES

REFERENCES

Boud D, Keogh R, Walker D 1985 Reflection: turning experience into learning. Kogan Page, London

Boyd EM, Fales AW 1983 Reflective learning: key to learning from experience. Journal of Humanistic Psychology 23: 99–117

Gibbs G 1988 Learning by doing: a guide to teaching and learning methods. Further Education Unit, Oxford Polytechnic, Oxford

Honey P, Mumford A 1992 The manual of learning styles, 3rd edn. Peter Honey, Maidenhead

Johns C 1994 Guided reflection. In: Palmer A, Burns S, Bulman C (eds) Reflective practice in nursing: the growth of the professional practitioner. Blackwell Science, Oxford

Kolb DA 1984 Experiential learning: experience as the source of learning and development. Prentice Hall, London, p 38

Malim T, Birch A (eds) 1998 Introductory psychology. Macmillan, Basingstoke, p 291

Nursing and Midwifery Council 2002 Code of professional conduct. NMC, London

Rolfe G 1996 Closing the theory practice gap: a new paradigm for nursing. Butterworth–Heinemann, Oxford, p 127

Schon D 1983 The reflective practitioner: how professionals think in action. Basic Books, New York

ACKNOWLEDGEMENTS

To Gail Alkins and Lisa Egerton, nursing students in the School of Health and Human Sciences, Liverpool John Moores University, for permission to use their reflective accounts.

3 Using the library

Sue Brain with Kym Martindale

KEY ISSUES

- Library resources and services
- Information resources
- Accessing library resources

- Electronic sources
- Literature searching
- Obtaining literature

INTRODUCTION

This chapter and Chapters 4, 5 and 8 are about gathering information from a variety of sources. The emphasis is on your role in the process – how you can make the material and resources work for you. Gathering information can be broadly divided into two stages:

- locating the material
- using the material.

This chapter deals with the first stage; Chapters 8 and 9 look in detail at the second.

The skills for finding the evidence and literature searching, together with skills to critically evaluate material, have received renewed emphasis in the light of clinical governance and clinical effectiveness (NHS Executive 1999), evidence-based health care (Sackett et al 1996). Literature-searching skills are a vital component of the evidence-based approach. Access to information has been transformed with the advent of the Internet, electronic publishing and the arrival of gateways such as the National Electronic Library for Health (NeLH). Therefore, familiarity with information technology (IT), a grasp of basic computer skills (see Chapter 4) and information searching skills are vital.

Learning is nowadays seen as a lifelong process and is no longer viewed as something that finishes with leaving school or college. Recent developments in the UK include the creation of the NHS University, with the explicit aim that the 'NHSU wants to put lifelong learning at the heart of better health and social care'. Library and information-gathering skills will be important throughout your working career and beyond.

CRITICAL PROCESS

Finding and using information is a process that involves critical thinking, understanding and constant interpretation. It is a questioning process and provides a good foundation for the reasoning skills you need to present a written argument (see Chapter 9).

Guiding principle – be clear about your purpose

Gathering information is done more effectively if you have defined your purpose. Whether you are deciding which database to search or which article to read, keep your purpose clearly in mind. For example, while preparing for an essay, keep the essay question clearly visible (a useful tip for when you come to write it) to prevent you from straying down interesting but irrelevant avenues. Information overload means that there is a huge amount of material available and it is easy to be overwhelmed. Knowing your purpose keeps you focused and enables others, e.g. library staff, to help you.

Information sources

As a student (and professional) you can expect to use the following:

- Libraries for:
    - books (general and specialized texts)
    - journals (also known as periodicals or serials; professional, academic or specialized)
    - audiovisual material (videos, multimedia packages)
    - reference material (dictionaries, directories, encyclopaedias, etc.)
- The Internet (access via the library or from home) for:
    - databases (MEDLINE, CINAHL, etc.)
    - publications (electronic or e-journals, government publications, etc.)
    - patient information (patient organization websites, newsgroups, etc.)
- Professional associations/specialist information centres for:
    - contacts
    - specialist information
    - patient information.

This chapter will concentrate on how to access the information sources generally found in libraries. The aim is not to turn you into an expert but to give you the confidence to use the expertise of the resources and staff.

LIBRARY RESOURCES AND SERVICES

Why use a library? Many people assume that nearly all the information they require is now available via the Internet. However it is still important to become familiar with the resources and services offered by libraries. It is true that many traditionally library-held resources (books, reports, journals, databases, etc.) are increasingly becoming available, and are easily accessible, online via the Internet. Most libraries would describe themselves as being in a hybrid situation at present, i.e. they hold both print and electronic resources.

It is important to remember that not all sources of information have been digitized yet and that access to traditional print resources is still necessary. Newer publications are increasingly being published both electronically and in print form. But there are still huge gaps in the literature, particularly in the earlier years, where information will only be available in print.

It is true that libraries are gradually moving away from the concept of being repositories and housing large physical collections of printed documents and journals. In the electronic age the librarian or information specialist's role is increasingly concerned with facilitating access and guiding users and researchers to the appropriate resources. We are facing an information explosion in all subject areas, and it can be difficult to know where to begin with your information gathering. Librarians, subject specialists, knowledge managers – they all have a role in offering guidance through the bewildering amount of information that exists, in whatever format – electronic, print, audio-visual, etc. Many libraries are developing their own portals or websites, which offer guidance to their users on which are the most useful and appropriate sources of information. These websites typically contain links to the library catalogue (also known as an open-access public catalogue, OPAC), user guides, other useful websites, listings of new resources and contact details. Try to find out whether your library has a website and add it to your Favorites or Bookmarks (depending on which Internet browser you use; this allows your web addresses to be saved so that they can easily be visited at a later time).

Library services

Here is a list of services typically offered by libraries. Your library may offer some or all of these:

- Loans service, reservations, short-term loans for items in heavy demand

- Open-access public catalogue (OPAC)
- Document delivery and interlibrary loans (access to resources held in other libraries)
- Enquiry facilities and subject-specialist librarians
- Registration and guidance on how to access specialist electronic resources
- Library website or portal
- Photocopying facilities
- Computers and printing facilities
- Quiet study space
- Laminators and binding facilities
- Video/DVD facilities
- Specialist IT and other equipment for students with visual impairment
- Current awareness and alerting services
- Training in literature searching and critical appraisal skills
- Induction sessions for new students
- Library guides and searching guides for specific databases or subject areas
- Specialist collections
- Outreach services – for example, in a hospital there may be a clinical librarian who gets involved in the ward rounds and who aims to provide quick and easy access to clinical information.

It is vital to get to know early on in your studies which services the library offers. These should be listed in the general library guide (available online or in print).

Resources

Most libraries will have the resources listed in the table below, which offer material appropriate to different search needs. How do you know which to use when, and how do you access them?

Table 3.1 gives a general picture of sources, means of access and purpose, but it is not meant to be exhaustive. Your own library may hold other resources.

You can probably begin to see how the type of information you need, i.e. your purpose, determines which source you use.

Take the two following questions, and, referring to Table 3.1 think (for about 5–10 minutes) where you would look for the material for the answer to each. There could be more than one source.

- Describe the structure and function of the skin
- What causes the skin condition psoriasis and how is it now treated?

TABLE 3.1	Resources typically available in a library	
Source	**Access**	**Purpose**
Books Textbooks Handbooks Research reports Government publications Theses Guidelines	Online public access catalogue (OPAC) listing Details of collections, shelf location and access information, e.g. shelf marks OPAC accessed via library workstation or library website (remote access, e.g. at home) Print, e-books and online	Core reading Background Context Factual Original research details and conclusions Policy documents Skills and guides Historical
Reference books Dictionaries Encyclopaedias Directories Yearbooks and almanacs Atlases Statistical publications (official and unofficial sources) Bibliographies	OPAC as above Print and online, e.g. Xrefer	Definitions Factual information Concise overviews Further reading or bibliographies Contacts Geography Population, socioeconomic and numerical data
Journals Research and popular Print and e-journals (also known as periodicals or serials)	OPAC as above or separate printed or on-line journal list gives titles, length of holding, location, access details Indexed – print or on-line indexes Internet databases with links to full text CD-ROM Internet	Current and specific material Current awareness Primary research papers Literature review articles News Information exchange Reviews Contacts Events Jobs
Newspapers Broadsheets Tabloids	OPAC as above or listed with journals as above Titles, length of holdings, location and access details	Current and contemporary Lay/popular material News and reports of latest research

(continued)

TABLE 3.1	(continued)	
Source	Access	Purpose
	Indexed	Reviews
	Print indexes	Factual
	Microfilm indexes	Statistics
	CD-ROM indexes	
	On-line indexes and full-text	
	on line	
	Print, CD-ROM or on line	
Audio-visual	OPAC as above for titles,	Instructive and learning
Videos or DVDs	holdings, location and access	packages
CD-ROMS		Factual
Audio tape or digital		Visual documentaries
Computerized assisted		TV programmes
learning (CAL) packages		Current and contemporary
Online e-learning packages		

Both questions deal broadly with the skin. The first concerns basic anatomy and physiology, factual information that is unlikely to change greatly. Textbooks and audiovisual material, i.e. videos, would probably provide excellent information for this question.

The second question deals with a specific skin condition and requires current information. Textbooks would provide some material and a medical dictionary would give an introductory definition, but you would need to use journal literature to discover the up-to-date treatment and care, and any research, findings or discussion/controversy concerning them. There might also be recent TV documentaries (recorded and held in the library) or relevant, current newspaper reports that might aid your understanding of the more clinical material in the health journals. Look for guidelines (e.g. Prodigy) and evidence-based summaries – e.g. Clinical Evidence (*British Medical Journal*), Bandolier, the Cochrane Library (systematic reviews).

WHAT RESOURCES DOES YOUR LIBRARY OFFER?

If you don't already know what your university and/or professional library holds, and where books and journals are kept and how you access electronic resources, find out! It's best to familiarize yourself with such things early in your course before you need them. All libraries should offer induction and tuition in the first few weeks of a course. Make the most of such opportunities – seek them out.

The library catalogue

This resource must be mastered as soon as possible. The catalogue tells you what stock the library has and where it is shelved. The type of material listed will depend on the library but will certainly include books and government publications. Audio-visual materials may well be in the catalogue but there may be a separate listing of journals and newspapers.

Nowadays, libraries have computerized catalogue access, often known as OPAC. OPACs can tell you what material the library holds by author, subject or title, where any item is shelved or whether it's out on loan. Other facilities are dependent on the system used by the library. It is worth bearing in mind that most university, college (and public) library catalogues are now accessible via the Internet, usually via the library's website.

JOURNAL LITERATURE

What is a journal?

Essentially, journals are the way you communicate with your fellow professionals nationally and internationally. All professions and trades have journals. The medical and health professions have thousands. From this you will deduce that your library will not have all of them; more on that later.

You may come across journals referred to as 'serials' and/or 'periodicals', because they are published periodically and because each issue is part of the whole. A journal may be published weekly, monthly, bi-monthly, quarterly (four times a year) or occasionally less frequently. Generally, the issues appearing in one year are described as one volume, each year having one volume number. The *Journal of Advanced Nursing* is an example of a research journal that is published twice a month and consists (unusually) of four volumes per year (24 issues) with each volume consisting of six parts or issues; for example, there were four volumes in 2003, volumes 41–44. The October 2003 volume started with volume 44 part 1. The standard way of writing this is 44(1). The volume number precedes the issue number, which is in brackets.

How is the material in journals different from that in books?

Journals differ from books in four important ways:

- **Currency**: books can take 2–4 years to reach publication; journal literature is usually published within months, depending on the frequency of the journal itself. Increasingly, journals are being published electronically via the Internet, making them even more immediately available.

- **Specificity**: articles are condensed material and are therefore focused on specific areas. When you search the literature, your subject headings can be correspondingly precise.

- **Ongoing**: reports of ongoing, long-term research projects are to be found in the relevant journals, information otherwise unavailable for perhaps years.

- **Contemporary**: literature from journals published in the 1960s, for example, directly reflects the tone, attitudes and knowledge of the time, unmuddied by hindsight.

What sort of material do the different journals contain?

You can expect the more frequent (weekly, monthly) journals to contain current affairs, jobs and listings, and articles that are informative, wide-ranging but not necessarily research-based. The name of the journal is a fair indication of its broad aim, standards and content. So, the *Nursing Times* or *Nursing Standard* aim to inform the nursing profession and will cover anything they consider relevant. The *Journal of Cancer Nursing* clearly has a narrower remit; articles are longer, specific and often research-based. Published bi-monthly, its material is less immediate and more analytical.

ACCESSING THE JOURNAL LITERATURE

When you need to find out whether a book contains information on a topic, you use the index at the back. This tells you if the topic is covered, on which pages and in how much detail. The principle is the same with journals, i.e. you use an index. It tells you what articles are available on a subject and in which journal you will find them. The chief difference is that journal indexes are generally published as electronic bibliographic databases; they also index many different journals simultaneously. Many databases provide links to the full text of selected electronic journals, e.g. services such as Thomson Dialog, Ovid, ProQuest, EBSCO, etc.

There are advantages to this. Remember that there are thousands of health and health-related journals, hundreds in nursing alone. If these were indexed individually instead of collectively, searching the literature would be an enormous task and you would be restricted to the journals your library held. (The flip side is that using journal bibliographic databases means you will probably require some articles not held by your library or linked to electronically; most libraries recognize this and will request articles from other sources via the interlibrary loans system.)

How much information does a database give about articles?

Index information consists of the basic bibliographic details about any one item. For a journal article these details should be:

- title of article
- author(s)
- journal name
- volume and part numbers
- date
- page numbers
- abstract (not always included)
- descriptors, subject headings.

This information makes up the citation or reference. Depending on the indexing service used, you may be told more about the article, e.g. how much further reading it includes or how many references it has cited, whether the content is research-based, statistical, etc.

Abstracts

Many databases provide a summary of content. This summary is called an abstract. Abstracts help you to make a more informed decision about the value to you of an article, paper or report. They are not a substitute for the original text and must not be treated as such. You must not quote them in your own writing as if you had read the original full-length work. In addition, the indexing terms (descriptors or subject headings) may also be listed. These are the terms used by the person who indexes items and may be useful in helping you to find similar articles.

ELECTRONIC DATABASES

Finding journal article citations used to involve searching through a printed index or abstracting publication. This was very labour-intensive and time-consuming. With the advent of CD-ROMs, and more recently the Internet, this task is made much easier, more flexible and much faster. Increasingly, electronic bibliographic databases are replacing the traditional indexing and abstracting services. The publishers of CD-ROMs and printed indexes now make their services available via the Internet, either by subscription services to institutions, or freely available, as in the case of PubMed (the free version of MEDLINE produced by the US National Library of Medicine). It is now possible to perform a literature search and gather source material from an integrated service such as Thomson Dialog, ProQuest or Ovid. Your library will probably have access to one or a number of similar services. These enable a search for citations to be run on various databases and from there to link directly to the full-text of journal articles.

Electronic databases allow you to search terms in combination, e.g. 'breast cancer' and 'case studies' and 'postoperative care'. Searching electronic databases gives you the advantage of more means of access to the information, and therefore greater control over your search. There are other benefits, including being able to print out your search results, e-mail or download them to disk or to reference management software, together with the added advantage of being able to access full-text articles in some cases. Again, find out now what your library offers and start using it!

As mentioned above, there are so many health journals and other types of health literature that no single bibliographic database can cover all the material published. Most are fairly comprehensive and cover a number of subject areas but are designed for specific disciplines, e.g. nursing and midwifery databases include CINAHL (Cumulative Index to Nursing and Allied Health Literature) and the BNI (British Nursing Index), MEDLINE and EMBASE cover biomedical subject areas, including nursing and midwifery, but have a stronger emphasis on clinical medicine.

It is your information needs that determine which indexes are best and when. Table 3.2 lists some of the databases available in the health information field, but there are many others. It is always advisable to run a literature search on several databases and not to rely solely on a single source. Despite some overlap between databases, different results will be produced. CINAHL and MEDLINE have some overlap but will also produce unique citations.

STARTING THE LITERATURE SEARCH

The first step in any literature search is to be clear about the meaning of the overall question and the meaning of the words or concepts contained within it. In other words, right from the very beginning it is essential that you are clear about what it is you are looking for.

TABLE 3.2   Some of the best known databases (most are available via the Internet or CD-ROM)

Name and producer	Access	Years covered	Description
MEDLINE US National Library of Medicine	PubMed (Internet with free access) NeLH – NHS National Core Content Clinical Databases Information aggregators, e.g. Thomson Dialog, Ovid	OLDMEDLINE 1953–1965 MEDLINE 1966– 'In process citations' are very new citations and provide basic citation information prior to receiving full indexing and MeSH headings	Indexes 4600 biomedical journals Medicine, nursing, midwifery, dentistry, veterinary medicine, health-care systems 14 million citations Bibliographic records, abstracts. Uses MeSH subject indexing International coverage
CINAHL (Cumulative Index to Nursing and Allied Health Literature)	CINAHL Direct Online Service NeLH – NHS National Core Content Clinical Databases	1982–	Indexes 1200 journals in nursing, midwifery and allied health Bibliographic records, with abstracts Uses CINAHL subject headings
EBSCO Information Services	Information aggregators, e.g. Thomson Dialog, Ovid		International coverage
EMBASE	Elsevier bibliographic database	1974–	A biomedical and pharmacological database with strong UK and European coverage
Elsevier	NeLH – NHS National Core Content Clinical Databases Information aggregators, e.g. Thomson Dialog, Ovid		Indexes 4000 journals 9 million citations Subject indexing using EMTREE (similar to MeSH). Some overlap with MEDLINE
BNI (British Nursing Index) Bournemouth University, Poole Hospital NHS Trust, Salisbury Health Care Trust, RCN	NeLH – NHS National Core Content Clinical Databases Information aggregators, e.g. Thomson Dialog, Ovid	1985–	Nursing, midwifery and community health-care database Bibliographic but does not include abstracts Indexes 220 journals UK coverage and updated monthly UK coverage

(continued)

TABLE 3.2	(continued)		
Name and producer	Access	Years covered	Description
AMED (Allied and Complementary Medicine Database) British Library	NeLH – NHS National Core Content Clinical Databases Information aggregators, e.g. Thomson Dialog, Ovid	1985–	Complementary medicine, palliative care, occupational therapy, physiotherapy, podiatry and rehabilitation, speech and language therapy Uses the AMED thesaurus of indexing terms Indexes nearly 600 journals
PscyINFO American Psychological Association	NeLH – NHS National Core Content Clinical Databases Information aggregators, e.g. Thomson Dialog, Ovid	1987–	Psychology and the psychological aspects of related disciplines, e.g. medicine, psychiatry, nursing, sociology, education, pharmacology, physiology, linguistics, anthropology, business and law Indexes 1500 journals
DH Data Department of Health Library (UK)	NeLH – NHS National Core Content Clinical Databases	1983–	Health service and hospital administration, NHS, nursing, primary care
ProQuest ProQuest Information and Learning	NeLH – NHS National Core Content Clinical Databases	Various dates	Three databases offering access to 1000 full-text journals: ProQuest Medical Library, Proquest Nursing Journals, ProQuest Psychology Journals
National Research Register Department of Health	Free access via the Internet	2000– Some records from 1990s	A database of ongoing and recently completed research projects funded by, or of interest to, the UK National Health Service Over 110000 records
ASSIA (Applied Social Sciences Index and Abstracts) Cambridge Scientific Abstracts	Cambridge Scientific Abstracts	1987–	312000 citations 650 journals US and UK Health, social services, psychology, sociology, economics, politics, race relations and education

You will need to return at intervals and remind yourself of the question. Successful searching depends on a careful analysis of the title, the choice of search terms and the way these are combined.

Often a good place to start is using dictionaries, encyclopaedias, subject handbooks, companions or textbooks to get a general grasp or overview of the topic. Doing a brief search on the Internet using a search engine or directory site may also help you to get an overview of the subject and may lead to some useful ideas to get you started. When answering a question, consider carefully which aspect or facet of a subject is being asked about. If you are responsible for setting an area to study yourself, narrow it down to a particular aspect if you find that your initial subject area is too large.

Are you working to a deadline? Leave enough time to plan, search for information, order materials if necessary, and read material. Don't forget, you still have to write your essay.

Consider your search/information needs

What sort of information do you need?

■ *Research: primary original research studies or secondary studies, i.e. material derived from the primary research – also consider whether qualitative or quantitative research is required*

■ *News reportage*

■ *Factual*

■ *Reviews/overviews of the literature*

■ *Opinion*

■ *Theory, ideas, philosophical perspective*

■ *Government policy or reports*

■ *Historical*

■ *Personal experience*

■ *Surveys or statistics*

■ *Practice guidelines (National Institute for Clinical Excellence, Royal Colleges, SIGN, Prodigy, etc.)*

Search terms

The first step is to break the question down into its main concepts. Have you thought about your search terms/subject headings? Think carefully about what headings you might use and how the thesauruses and indexing terms might express your subject. It is useful to brainstorm this, creating a spider map of your subject area. This helps to identify specific and broad terms, and provides a rough, visual hierarchy of the subject.

Limits

You also need to decide on the limitations to apply to the search. Think about how you might want to limit your search by:

- *age group – neonate, infant, child, adolescent, adult, elderly*
- *study group (human or animal)*
- *gender*
- *language*
- *publication date – within the past year, 2 years, 5 years, 10 years or further back?*
- *country – international or specific country?*
- *publication type – clinical trial, review, etc.*

Most databases have the facility to limit in some way, such as year (e.g. publications published within the last 5 years) or enable you to search on specific journal titles. They may also enable you to search by study type, e.g. clinical trial, review, etc.

Evidenced-based healthcare and clinical questions

When asking questions that relate to clinical questions it is worth considering a number of aspects.

Think about the way you ask the question. PICO is the recommended method of framing your question:

P – Patient/population
I   – Intervention or exposure
C – Comparison: intervention/no intervention
O – Outcomes.

The next step is to consider whether you are looking at therapy, diagnosis, prognosis or aetiology questions. Various search strategies can be employed for searching the literature; these include search filters. PubMed Clinical Filters is an example of a service with predefined filters that enable you to type in search terms, indicate the category and specify the emphasis on either a sensitive search (broad) or specific search (specific). SUMsearch offers a similar search facility with predefined choices for search emphasis provided. Further information may be found at the ADEPT website (ScHARR). The websites of the Centre for Evidence-based Medicine, based at Oxford, and the Centre for Evidence-based Medicine, University of Toronto, contain useful information on conducting evidence-based searching and the skills of critical appraisal.

Research study types or the hierarchy of evidence/levels of evidence are important when considering clinical questions. The highest level, 1, is normally a systematic review (the Cochrane Library being a prime source) while level 2 includes well-conducted randomized-controlled trials, right down to level 5, which is expert opinion. See the websites mentioned above for further information.

Being aware of these considerations is helpful before attempting a clinical search for information. The type of research study, its methodology and design, and its applicability to your practice are all important considerations in evidence-based healthcare. *How to Read a Paper* (Greenhalgh and Taylor 2001), published by the *British Medical Journal*, with chapters from the 1997 edition available via the BMJ website, is also worth reading.

Which database?

You will have realized by now that your search needs dictate your choice of database or resource used! The exercise below (maximum 10 minutes needed) gives you some practice at this.

This exercise involves matching search needs to the right database. Using Table 3.2, decide which database might be most appropriate for finding the necessary material for the search questions below. There is no right or wrong choice exactly but, clearly, some databases are better than others.

As you match search and databases, note the reasons for the choices you have made. This may help to clarify the thinking behind your decision.

1. What effect does a hip replacement have on patients' self-image, and how might that influence their recovery?
2. Does nurse education equip students to cope with the emotional stress of nursing terminally ill patients?
3. What, if any, relation is there between inequality in health and social class?

I   This question encompasses two issues: the psychological and social effects – psychosocial factors – of a condition, and the role of the carer in recognizing and dealing with these effects. There is a clear nursing angle, so the indexes CINAHL or BNI would all be useful sources. A combined search of CINAHL under hip surgery and self-image (or whatever the correct search terms might be) would swiftly reveal what, if any, material is available.

The nursing indexes are the obvious source for the caring angle. However, you might want to read current material on the subject of self-concept, and explore its psychology. PsycLIT would then be a useful source.

It is probably immaterial whether the articles you find are American, British or Australian, as there is no particular cultural slant to the search. Your main concern is the subject, which is universal.

2   Again, this is clearly a nursing issue. CINAHL or BNI would be appropriate routes to the relevant material. However, the question is also about stress, death and education. The educational element needs you to be aware of the country of origin of the material you might find; it could well still be relevant for the sake of contrast or proposed change, but if you require only UK material use the UK indexes first.

You could search MEDLINE for information on how effective medical education is in this regard. General material on occupational stress can be found in any of the sources mentioned, but add DH Data for a management angle.

3   This question is primarily sociological. A database with sociological content, e.g. ASSIA, would be an appropriate source. DH Data or the Health Management Information Consortium (HMIC) might provide information on monitoring the quality of the delivery of health across society. Again, the country of origin might be important, although American, etc., material could be useful for comparison.

Which search terms?

Having identified the appropriate database, you need to clarify your search terms or subject headings. These are the words you use to look up your subject in the databases. They may also be referred to as keywords.

Identifying your search terms happens in two stages:

1   Highlighting the key terms (or main concepts) in your essay question
2   Ensuring that they are the terms used by the databases you intend to search.

For the first stage, look again at the questions in the exercise above.

Take 10 minutes to identify what you consider to be the keywords for the search (then check them against those below).

1. hip replacement; self-image; recovery

2. nurse education; students; stress; terminally ill

3. inequality; health: social class.

It is possible that your keywords are not exactly the same as those used by any of the databases you intend searching.

It is helpful at this stage to spend a few minutes brainstorming for alternatives. Alternative terms/keywords:

1. hip replacement: hip surgery/hip prosthesis/artificial hip; self-image: body-image/self-concept/self-esteem; recovery: rehabilitation/postoperative care.

It is also likely that, in some cases, the terms you use will be different depending on the database, despite the fact that you're looking up the same subject.

These differences are due to cultural differences, terminology, spelling and diversity of language. For example, look at the two lists in Box 3.1, both full of terms related to their subject.

BOX 3.1	*Cancer*	*Ageing*
	Cancer	Ageing/aging
	Oncology	Aged
	Neoplasm	Elderly
	Tumour/tumor	Old age
	Growth	Geriatric
	Carcinosis	Gerontology
	Melanoma	Older person/people

A database could use quite a different term to the one you have chosen to search. If your search terms do not match the database you are using then you are wasting your time. If you search for geriatric nursing and find no material, there are two possible explanations:

- there may not be anything published/available
- the database has used the indexing term 'care of the elderly'.

But, how do you know which explanation is the true one?

It is essential when you are searching a database that you speak its language, even allowing for electronic databases' increased flexibility over the printed index. Some databases automatically convert your free-text or natural language terms into the subject terms or key-words of that database. This is known as 'mapping'.

Most databases try to help by providing a list of their terms for you to check before you begin to search. Called a thesaurus, or sub-ject headings list, this has two functions:

- to provide you with the correct search terms for that database (see first entry in Box 3.2)

- to introduce you to narrower (more specific), related or broader search terms, i.e. to alert you to other headings, which may be equally or more relevant (see second entry in Box 3.2).

BOX 3.2	*Thesaurus entries*

	Nurse education
	    see Education, nursing
	Education, nursing
	    see *also*
	    Education, nursing, Baccalaureate
	    Education, nursing, continuing
	    Education, nursing, post-registration

Such a list is essential, not only to you, the searcher, but also to those compiling the database. They need to standardize their headings so that related material is clustered under the same term, ensuring that you will find all the material available on a subject. Every year new subject terms are added; this reflects the growth of information, the need for more specific terms and the changing language. Consulting a database's thesaurus or list of keywords informs you of the best search terms for that database. If your terms are wrong you will not find the material. Subject headings/search terms are really key words.

MeSH (Medical Subject Headings) is the MEDLINE thesaurus and is available on the MEDLINE website. MeSH is an example of a controlled language with a very well-defined structure, e.g. the MeSH tree structure.

When you find useful references as a result of a database search it is worth looking at the descriptors or indexing terms that have been used. You can then refine your search terms to incorporate these into your search as appropriate.

A thesaurus or subject headings list is not infallible. It won't always list your original search term and therefore alternatives. In this instance, you need to be your own thesaurus. This is where brainstorming possible subject headings is helpful. Another source of help is, of course, the librarian.

Use the following steps:
- Identify your search terms from your essay question, or write down your search need in a way that helps you to highlight the keywords. Brainstorm for alternative keywords/search terms.

- Browse the database's list of indexing terms or use the thesaurus; it ensures you are using the correct search terms and those most appropriate to your search.
- Be aware of variations in American and UK spellings and allow for these.
- Identifying your search terms properly will retrieve relevant material, or confirm its absence.

SEARCHING ELECTRONIC DATABASES

Mastering a few basic search techniques, such as how to use Boolean operators, will prove invaluable when searching electronic databases. These techniques may also be applied when using Internet search engines. Some search engines allow quite sophisticated search techniques to be used, similar to the methods used when searching databases. Wherever possible it is advisable to spend some time looking at the search help pages. Most databases or Internet search engines include a help facility. The library may have prepared a user guide to searching specific databases, which is either printed or available online. These will contain useful tips and enable you to get the most out of the source being used.

Boolean operators

Using Boolean operators offers more control and the ability to refine searches. The main operators are AND, OR, NOT. Plan how the concepts are going to be linked in your search statement. Use Boolean logic to narrow, widen or exclude when combining terms. Link your terms by using AND to narrow, OR to widen or NOT to exclude terms.

- AND is used to narrow a search statement. This ensures that all the search terms appear on the web page or document, e.g. cancer AND lung AND patient AND nursing results in all of these terms appearing in the citations retrieved.

- OR is often used to widen a search. Using OR between words, e.g. nursing OR nurse results in either one or both words appearing in the reference. It enables you to specify more than one word, term, phrase or synonym in a search statement, e.g. cancer OR neoplasm OR tumour OR tumor. It is useful, for instance, where a database includes both American and UK spellings.

- NOT enables the exclusion of a word or phrase from a search statement. Combining terms with NOT, e.g. child NOT adult means that the first word must be present but not the second.

- Proximity searching with NEAR or WITH or ADJACENT is often used to specify how close terms should appear to each other, e.g. palliative NEAR care. It is possible to specify that words should appear within the same sentence or paragraph.

Truncation and wild cards

Using a truncation symbol such as *, ? or $ after or within a word enables you to pick up words with a variety of spellings. Many words have a common stem or root, which can be used as a search term. Using a truncation symbol allows you to broaden the search to include all records that contain any variation of the stem. This is particularly useful where you are unsure of the exact spelling, when including plurals or where there may be alternative spellings.

- Using hospital* will find references with the words hospitals, hospitalisation, hospitalization, hospitalized, etc.
- nurs* will find nurse, nurses, nursing, etc.

Some databases allow truncation or wild card symbols to be used in the middle of words or at the beginning of a word.

- wom*n will find the words woman or women;
- *ye* will find stye, styes, eye, eyes, etc.

Use these symbols with caution, particularly where a word might appear quite frequently in a database. It will slow the computer down when searching and may result in a large number of irrelevant items being found!

Nesting

Nesting, or the use of parentheses – or brackets () – allows complex queries to be constructed. The brackets indicate the order in which the logical operators or commands are to be carried out by a computer. These are used with multiple Boolean commands and need careful planning, e.g. (child OR infant) AND (cancer OR tumour*) AND pain control. The terms in brackets will be searched as queries in their own right, one at a time, before being linked to the phrase pain. Without the use of the parentheses confusion would ensue and irrelevant results would be found.

How useful is that reference?

It is difficult to deduce the potential value of an article from the basic information given in a database, i.e. the citation. However, there are indicators:

- Is there an abstract?
- Check the authors' credentials – they may be well-known in their field and have written other material.

- Is the journal cited academic, scholarly, research-based or more news-based?
- How long is the article? If long, consider the time necessary to read and understand it; if short, how informative will it be?
- How many references does it cite? These may lead to other material on your subject and may indicate the authenticity of the author/s' work.
- What type of paper is being cited? Is it original research or a review of the literature? Is it a systematic review, meta-analysis or randomized controlled trial? Where does it fit into the hierarchy of evidence?
- Is the article itself cited by others? Check a citation index if possible (ask your library staff); this will tell you if, and how often, this particular article has been referred to by other published authors.
- Ask tutors and fellow students or colleagues if they have read, seen or know of a certain work or author.
- Practise critically appraising the article and considering the applicability and appropriateness of research results (see section on evidence-based healthcare).

Judging the relevance of an article is a skill, which will come with practice. You will make mistakes because you cannot be 100% certain of any material until you have read it. There won't always be an abstract, authors and journals are numerous and many will be unknown to you. But, if your search terms are accurate and well thought-out, you are more likely to retrieve relevant material.

THE INTERNET

The Internet is an increasingly important resource for anyone undertaking research. It makes information available to a wide audience at a relatively low cost. It has had a tremendous impact on the provision of health information both for professionals and the public alike, and it is developing at a phenomenal pace. Access to the Internet is via the library or from home. Your library will probably provide help with searching the Internet. It will also provide you with the means – registration (providing you with a username and password) – to access specialist online resources, e.g. databases and online full-text journals, subscribed to by your college or institution.

Internet resources

Many resources traditionally available through a library are now accessible via the Internet. These include newspapers, journals, databases (as already mentioned), encyclopaedias, dictionaries, some books and atlases, government publications (such as policy documents and reports), statistical data, drug information and patient leaflets. Using the Internet is not a substitute for using a good library. With regard to research material it lacks the coverage, depth and span of holdings that a good library can provide, but it is still a useful adjunct or starting point for research.

The Internet contains information from a wide range of bodies, including educational establishments, government departments, institutions, societies, companies, voluntary organizations, professional organizations, the media, health consumer groups and individuals. The main problem centres on its democratic, but unregulated, nature. As already mentioned, quality and reliability of information is a major concern and you must always bear this in mind when using Web sources (see Chapter 8). The principles established by tools such as HON (Health on the Net Foundation), CHIQ (Centre for Health Information Quality) and Discern (developed to assess the quality of consumer health publications) are worth bearing in mind when using web-based sources. A degree of caution is required when using the Internet and it is important to consider the reputation of the originator of the content and whether commercial or other interests are involved.

Finding information on the Internet

Health information gateway sites

It is advisable to start your Internet search using a reputable gateway website. These sites contain links to resources that have been either evaluated or quality-checked. The UK National Electronic Library for Health (NeLH) is being developed, with librarian involvement, as an NHS gateway for UK health professionals and aims to provide easy access to best current knowledge and know-how, with the aim of improving health and health care, clinical practice and patient choice. The NeLH homepage has links to key resources such as:

- The Cochrane Library
- Clinical Evidence (BMJ)
- NeLH Guidelines Finder
- Prodigy
- The National Institute for Clinical Excellence
- MIDIRS resources
- UK National Service Frameworks
- The British National Formulary (BNF)

- Protocols and care pathways
- Clinical databases (UK users via Athens)
- Full-text journals (UK users via Athens)
- Medical dictionaries
- Specialist libraries (by subject and profession – nurse, midwife, child health, cancer, health management, etc.)
- Hitting the Headlines (critically appraised news stories)
- OMNI-reviewed Internet resources and NMAP Internet resources for nursing and midwifery and allied health professions.

There is a search facility, although this does not search all NeLH resources in depth.

From NeLH there are other useful links, including the NHS Direct website, which provides information for the public. There is a health encyclopaedia, a self-help guide, hot topics, a search service for local NHS services, frequently asked questions (FAQs) and an online enquiry service.

NeLH includes a link to NMAP. This grew out of a website called Nursing and Health Care Resources on the Net, compiled by Rod Ward, a lecturer at Sheffield University. It evaluates and categorizes Internet resources under headings and gives each site a description. NMAP acts as a useful gateway website for nurses and midwives.

There are similar US equivalents. The US National Library of Medicine has a Health Information page containing links to MED-LINEPlus, MEDLINE/PubMed and the US National Library of Medicine (NLM) Gateway (provides cross-searching of NLM resources). MEDLINEPlus, produced by the NLM, aims to link the public to the most reliable and authoritative information. It has a comprehensive medical encyclopaedia; a medical dictionary; a health topics section covering over 600 topics with links to resources produced by authoritative bodies, institutes and organizations; news; directories and other resources. Healthfinder is another gateway developed by the US Department of Health and Human Services. It has links to evaluated health information for the general public. HealthInsite is the Australian equivalent, providing quality-assessed information originating from a variety of sources. Sections cover lifestyle; conditions and diseases; life stages and events; population groups; expert groups.

Evaluating health information on the Internet

There are a number of evaluation tools, codes, kitemarking schemes and evaluation tools for assessing the validity of Internet health information. One of the original codes is the Health on the Net Foundation

(HoN), a not-for-profit Geneva-based organization that has developed a code of conduct for health websites. These eight guidelines cover aspects such as authority, confidentiality and transparency of sponsorship. Its website includes a medical search engine, MedHunt, a medical documents finder and HONselect, a medical search engine that uses MeSH headings. There are other criteria, codes and kitemarking schemes for evaluating Internet resources, e.g. OMNI/BIOME criteria, Discern, Hi Quality, Judge: websites for Health, the Canadian Health Network, MedCIRCLE.

Internet search engines

Search engines allow you to type in keywords to search the World Wide Web. They act as indexes to the vast amount of information available on the Web. A word of caution, though, as they may lead you to totally misleading and inaccurate information! You need to develop skills to evaluate the results produced by search engines. Search engines employ robots or 'spiders' to trawl the net for new content and then index words from the pages they find into vast databases. Typing in keywords enables you to search an index of websites. Even the best of these is only able to index a limited percentage of the rapidly growing web content. One of the best-known search engines is Google. Others include AllTheWeb and Alta Vista. See Search Engine Watch for the latest information and reviews on search engines.

For general Internet searching advice and tutorials see the tutorial *Finding Information on the Internet: A Tutorial*, produced by the Teaching Library at the University of California at Berkeley, or the Resources Discovery Network (RDN) Virtual Training Suite.

When using a search engine, remember to look at the search help pages. These contain useful tips to give you more control over your searching. For instance, when searching for phrases, or where you are searching for words that must occur together, enclose the search terms in double quotation marks, e.g. "Tourette's syndrome". Some search engines, such as Alta Vista's advanced search facility, allow you to use Boolean operators or to restrict searches in some way, e.g. to words in the titles of websites, or to search for academic sites or educational websites only.

Directories are hierarchically arranged databases of websites with a search facility. They categorize websites under subject headings. They are compiled by human beings and are therefore more selective than the general search engines, and are useful for finding specialist websites. Yahoo is a long-established, well-known directory site. Other similar sites include LookSmart. Most search engines (such as Google) now include a directory as part of their service.

Metasearch engines search a number of search engines or directories at the same time and attempt to retrieve the most relevant results for you. They are useful for getting an overall feel for a subject. Not all search engines use the same search syntax so, having searched using a metasearch engine you are then better using a single search engine and using its syntax to fine-tune the search. Vivisimo is an example of an interesting search engine that clusters results into related groupings.

General subject gateways can be invaluable in directing you to evaluated resources on the World Wide Web. These act as gateways or subject guides and contain links to high-quality resources, which are useful for research purposes. They generally include descriptions of websites and are compiled and hosted by educational institutions. NeLH has already been mentioned as a health information gateway but general academic gateways include the Resource Discovery Network (RDN).

Evidence-based health care

A good starting place for finding evidence-based resources, after NeLH, is Netting the Evidence, produced by the School of Health and Related Research at Sheffield University (ScHARR). This contains links to some invaluable resources and is regularly updated. The TRIP database is freely available for searching and its search technology underpins the NeLH search facility. TRIP+ is the premium service available via subscription. TRIP was created in 1997 to bring together all the 'evidence-based' healthcare resources available on the Internet.

Journals

As previously mentioned, many research journals are available through services such as Dialog, Ovid, ProQuest, EBSCO or Ingenta. Many journals arc also available electronically, via their publishers' websites. Many make contents pages, together with abstracts, or selected articles from the current issue freely available e.g. the *Nursing Standard* or *Nursing Times*. Some, such as the *British Medical Journal* make the full contents of the current issue and back issues freely available, together with a search facility. Many operate free alerting services that help you stay in touch with the latest contents of that particular title. A good source of free medical journals is a website simply called Free Medical Journals.

Databases

The US National Library of Medicine launched its free PubMed database service (MEDLINE) on the World Wide Web in 1997. It is directed at both health professionals and consumers and gives access to one of the premier biomedical databases, with records dating back to the 1950s. Currently there are over 14 million citations or references in this database. Its covers the biomedical sciences, including medicine and nursing. Access to the majority of databases is still mediated by your library, either on CD-ROM or on line via a subscription services (Ovid, Dialog, etc.). These require you to register and acquire a username and password. The library will be able to advise on registration and access requirements.

Newspapers and news services

Most newspapers, both national and local, have websites. Many provide access to their daily content and some have a limited search or archive facility. These sites do not provide total access to their contents, nor do they have a comprehensive search facility (as with a CD-ROM or an online subscription version). Nevertheless, they are still useful for finding news stories or for providing an overview of the daily news. Newspapers from around the world are available via such services as The Paperboy. General news services abound, including specialist health news services – Reuters, Ananova, BBC, CNN Health News.

Library catalogues

Most universities and colleges, and some professional societies and associations, make their library catalogues available via the Web. The HERO website (Higher & Research Opportunities in the United Kingdom) has links to the UK library OPACs in higher education. There is free access through the Consortium of University Research Libraries (COPAC) to the unified catalogues of some of the largest university research libraries in the UK and Ireland. The records include books and periodicals (but not periodical contents). The British Library, a national deposit library, provides a facility to search its catalogue (both reference and lending collections) on the Web. The Royal College of Nursing (RCN) library database is available online and includes references to books, journal articles (from 1985), theses and videos. Currently the Royal College of Midwives catalogue is not available on line, although an alternative freely available resources via NeLH is the MIDIRS database.

Access to these catalogues is useful for checking references and you should be able to request books from other libraries through your local library interlibrary loan system (check with your library).

Government and official publications

The UK Online.gov.uk website offers a useful gateway to government departments and publications. The UK Department of Health (DoH) website has to be a good starting point for anyone needing government publications. It contains COIN – a database containing DoH circulars – and POINT – a database that gives details and access to full text (where available) of departmental publications, including white papers. Many health-related publications can be found at The Stationery Office UK Official Publications on the Internet. They can be viewed by date, title or department. Acts of Parliament and other government department publications are now published on the Internet. Parliamentary publications, including Hansard (the daily debates), public and private bills and select committee publications, can be accessed in full at the UK Parliament website.

Statistics

The most obvious starting point for finding statistics is the Office for National Statistics (ONS) website. ONS is the government agency responsible for gathering and publishing statistical data. The Department of Health contains statistics and surveys on its websites. This includes data on public health, health care, social care, the workforce and expenditure. Other guides to health statistics on the Internet include Health Statistics: A Guide to Printed and Online Resources (London South Bank University). This contains numerous links to useful documents and websites.

USING OTHER LIBRARIES

It may become necessary to extend your search for material to other libraries that house specialist collections or resources your library does not hold. The Royal College of Nursing (telephone number 0207 409 3333, or see the RCN website) has its own library, including specialist historical and nursing research collections. Only RCN members and students attending courses at the RCN Institute are eligible to borrow items. Non-members can use the library for a charge and should contact the staff before visiting. The Royal College of Midwives (telephone number 0207 312 3535) also has a library. In order to use this you have to make an appointment.

The King's Fund Library (telephone number 0207 307 2568/2569 or see the website) welcomes visits from the public as well as enquiries in writing or by telephone or e-mail. It specializes in health management and policy. The library is reference only and this means that you will be unable to borrow material. As with most specialist libraries it is advisable to phone in advance to check opening hours and to make an appointment to visit.

The British Library is the national library and receives publications by legal deposit. It is split into a number of different collections. The St Pancras site includes the humanities reference collection together with the science, technology and business collections. It is available to those whose research needs cannot be adequately met by other libraries. Access is restricted and certain criteria have to be met. Contact the Reader Admissions Office (telephone number 0207 412 7000) or see the website for details.

In order to access libraries at other universities and colleges you will need to telephone in advance. You will only be allowed to use these at the discretion of the library staff if you are not a registered student at that institution.

Public libraries make access to their reference collections freely available, although to borrow items you have to study, work or be resident in the local authority's area. Reference collections are usually located in large central libraries and offer access to special collections such as local studies material. They usually house a wide range of encyclopaedias, dictionaries, directories, yearbooks, journals, reports and government and statistical publications. They may also provide Internet access and access to CD-ROM databases. You may have to book in advance to use special facilities such as CD-ROMs, microfiche/film viewers or the Internet. It is always a good idea to phone in advance if you want to use these facilities.

WHAT IF YOU FIND LITTLE OR NOTHING?

Information retrieval is a frustrating business. There will be times when there appears to be nothing published on your subject – nothing that answers your need. And it is also true that failure to locate any material can never be attributed with certainty to the fact that there is nothing. There will always be a niggling doubt that you didn't seek hard enough, or for long enough, in the right places; that the very item you require exists somewhere. This is when you have fallen prey to the myth 'I've thought of it, therefore it exists'.

Certainly, there will be times when you have to accept the awful truth and readjust your search (or do some research and get it published to fill the gap!). But don't give up straight away: first, be resourceful and adaptable in the following ways:

■ Check your search terms – use the thesaurus, library staff or fellow students

- Make sure you are using the most appropriate source – appropriate database, textbook vs journals, general vs specialist libraries/ information centres
- Is there comparable information available? For example, in the activity on page 63, question 1 could use research material from studies on breast cancer or AIDS – the key element is the patient's self-perception and response to their condition
- Talk to colleagues, fellow students, tutors and library staff – they have expertise, contacts and knowledge not available via established channels.

Box 3.3 contains a checklist that condenses the main points of this chapter and the steps of a literature search.

BOX 3.3

Preparation

1. Define your purpose: why do you need this information and what precisely do you need? Write this out.
2. Plan your time: allow for search setbacks, for obtaining items from elsewhere and for reading the material.
3. Familiarize yourself with your library's facilities and services as soon as possible – opening hours, catalogue, CD-ROM and Internet access, photocopiers, journals in stock, procedures for requesting items.

Defining your search

1. Identify your keywords from your search statement/essay question.
2. Brainstorm your keywords for alternative headings.
3. Identify appropriate sources.

Ask for help at any point.

Starting the search

1. Check your search terms in the subject headings list/thesaurus for each database or index you use.
2. Record the search terms you used and the sources searched, e.g. BNI 1999 under nurse education or CINAHL 1998–2000 under education–nursing and death–education. This saves you repeating parts of your search and can inform library staff in giving you further help. Electronic databases generally allow you to print or save your search, giving you an excellent record of what terms were used and how, i.e. your search strategy. You may have access and be able to download references directly into bibliographic management software such as EndNote, Procite or Reference Manager. This enables you to capture references from a wide range of sources, to insert them into documents and produce bibliographies with ease.
3. Record the full citation details of items, articles, etc. that you wish to locate and read. This information is necessary for swift location and for your own final reference list. Noting each citation separately on index cards enables easy filing with space for annotation, i.e. brief notes on its usefulness and content.

4. Locate/order and read your material, noting further search needs and ideas.

5. Adapt your search as necessary – modify search terms, explore related subject areas, use comparable material. This is developing your strategy. Record such developments.

6. Stick to your time plan and your purpose. Literature searching is time-consuming and full of distractions. Your time for searching and reading is limited. Be realistic and have a clear cut-off point (although you can note items of interest for another time).

There are twists and turns in the literature search, but you are not alone. You're not expected to struggle on without help. Professional help and expertise is to hand – use it! But help the professionals to help you by being clear about your purpose, your information need.

- Get to know your library and its resources
- Ask for help whenever you need it
- Make full use of any library tuition
- Allow time for library and literature searches
- Identify your information needs
- Define and stick to your purpose
- Your best sources of information will change according to your needs
- Spelling and terminology differ according to origin and source
- Journals contain much more current material than textbooks
- Your library is unlikely to hold everything you will need
- Your library can obtain material from other libraries
- Allow time to order material
- Keep references and records
- Practise these skills

CONCLUSION

In this chapter we have discussed and tested the process of information finding. At all stages, you have had to make decisions based on your needs, acting critically and reflectively. In order to do so, you have had to keep your purpose to the fore. The growth of electronic information sources, particularly the rapid development of the Internet and the World Wide Web, is markedly improving access to information. There is an enormous range of information available to you via libraries and the Internet. In Chapter 5 we will see how knowing your purpose also applies to using the information you acquire during your studies.

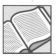

CHAPTER RESOURCES

GLOSSARY

Abstract: summary of the contents of a journal article, research paper, conference report or book.

Audiovisual: non-print items that need to be viewed or heard, such as videos or audiotapes. Sometimes known as media.

Bibliographic: relating to the details of the book or article. Bibliographical information, e.g. title, author, publication date, volume number, page numbers, etc. is necessary for the location of the item.

Boolean operators: logical operators (AND, OR, NOT) used to link keywords or search terms when searching a database.

CD-ROM: compact-disk read only memory. A computer-read disk with the capacity to store an enormous amount of digital data. DVD (digital versatile disk) has an even greater capacity to store data.

Citation: the giving of bibliographical information.

Current awareness: bulletins that provide information on recently published journal articles, books, reports, etc.

Database: a collection of, for example, bibliographic electronic records accessible via CD-ROM, online or Internet.

Index (journals): list of articles by subject.

Internet: a network linking millions of computers across the world and making vast amounts of information available from these computers.

Journals: regular publications (e.g. monthly, weekly, bi-monthly) that act as a forum for newly published research, news, articles and the professional exchange of information.

Literature search: search of mainly journal and research literature for material relating to a topic.

Online: live database, journal, etc. which is constantly being updated.

OPAC: (online public access catalogue). System that makes library catalogues accessible via a computer and replaces card catalogues.

Periodical: *see* Journals.

Reference: unit of bibliographical information.

Search engine: a computer program that enables the user to search the World Wide Web using keywords. Search engines index documents on the Web and compile vast databases of Web content, which are searchable.

Serial: *see* Journals.

Thesaurus: list of subject headings or indexing terms used by an index or database. It will often show the hierarchical relationship between terms, e.g. broader, narrower and related terms.

Website: a location on the World Wide Web, usually containing a home page and other pages, documents or files. It is compiled or managed by an individual organization or company.

World Wide Web: Consists of documents or pages written in a special language known as hypertext mark-up language (html). This enables links to be made to other documents and it supports graphics, audio and video files.

Internet sites

Ananova: www.ananova.com
ADEPT: www.shef.ac.uk/~scharr/ir/adept
AlltheWeb: www.alltheweb.com
AltaVista: www.altavista.com
BBC news: news.bbc.co.uk
British Library: www.bl.uk
British Medical Journal: www.bmj.com
Canadian Health Network: www.Canadian-health-network.ca
Centre for Evidence-Based Medicine (University of Oxford):
    www.cebm.net
Centre for Evidence-based Medicine (University of Toronto):
    www.cebm.utoronto.ca
CNN: www.cnn.com
Consortium of University Research Libraries (COPAC):
    www.copac.ac.uk/copac
Department of Health: www.dh.gov.uk
Discern: www.discern.org.uk
Finding Information on the Internet: a Tutorial (University College
    Berkeley Library): www.lib.berkeley.edu/TeachingLib/Guides/
    Internet/ FindInfo.html
Free Medical Journals: www.frccmedicaljournals.com
Google: www.google.com
Healthfinder: www.healthfinder.gov
Health on the Net Foundation: www.hon.ch
HealthInsite: www.healthinsite.gov.au
Health Statistics: A Guide to Printed and Online Resources
    (London South Bank University): www.lisa.sbu.ac.uk/resources/
    subjects/hsocc/ healthstats.html
HERO: www.hero.ac.uk/niss/niss_library4008.cfm
Hi Quality: www.hiquality.org.uk
How to Read a Paper – Trisha Greenhalgh, Rod Taylor:
    bmj.bmjjournals.com/collections/read.htm
Ingenta: www.ingenta.com
Judge: Websites for health: www.judgehealth.org.uk
King's Fund: www.kingsfund.org.uk
Looksmart: www.search.looksmart.com
MedCIRCLE: www.europa.eu.int/information_society/
    programmes/iap/projects/filtering/medcircle/index_en.htm

MIDIRS: www.midirs.org
National Electronic Library for Health (NeLH): www.nelh.nhs.uk
NLM Gateway: gateway.nlm.nih.gov/gw/Cmd
Netting the Evidence (ScHARR): www.shef.ac.uk/~scharr/ir/netting
NHS Direct: www.nhsdirect.nhs.uk
NHS University: www.nhsu.nhs.uk
NMAP: nmap.ac.uk
Nursing Standard: www.nursing-standard.co.uk
Nursing Times: www.nursingtimes.net
Office for National Statistics: www.statistics.gov.uk
OMNI (Organising Medical Networked Information): omni.ac.uk
Paperboy: www.thepaperboy.com.au/uk
Pinakes: www.hw.ac.uk/libWWW/irn/pinakes/pinakes.html
PubMed: www.ncbi.nlm.nih.gov/entrez/query.fcgi?db=PubMed
RDN Virtual Training Suite: www.vts.rdn.ac.uk
Resource Discovery Network: www.rdn.ac.uk
Reuters: www.reutershealth.com/en/index.html
Royal College of Midwives: www.rcm.org.uk
Royal College of Nursing: www.rcn.org.uk
Search Engine Watch: www.searchenginewatch.com
The Stationery Office UK Official Publications on the Internet:
    www.official-documents.co.uk
SUMsearch: sumsearch.uthscsa.edu
TRIP: www.update-software.com/scripts/clibNG/HTML/
    TRIPUsernameLogon.htm
UK Online: www.ukonline.gov.uk
UK Parliament: www.parliament.uk
Vivisimo: www.vivisimo.com
Yahoo: www.yahoo.com

REFERENCES

Greenhalgh T, Taylor R 2001 How to read a paper: the basics of evidence based medicine. BMJ Books, London
NHS Executive 1999 Clinical governance: quality in the new NHS. Department of Health, London
Sackett DL, Rosenberg WMC, Gray IAM, Richardson WS 1996 Evidence-based medicine: what it is and what it isn't. British Medical Journal 312: 71–72

4 Using information technology

Denis Anthony

KEY ISSUES

- **Data Protection Act**
- *Searching the Internet*
- *Applications: spreadsheets, statistics packages,*
- *qualitative analysis packages, bibliographic packages*
- *Reference management*
- **Systematic reviews**

INTRODUCTION

This chapter gives an overview of the common information technology (IT) applications that you may find useful as a research-aware clinical nurse keen to keep your clinical practice evidence-based. IT is also useful for managers, educators and researchers; all areas relevant to nursing.

Information technology can help you in your studies and enable you to use your study time more effectively. Although more and more nursing students at pre- and postregistration level have access to and understanding of computers and information technology, this chapter is aimed at the student who has little experience with computers. Those of you with some experience in using computers to help your studies will probably be able to skim quickly through some parts of this chapter.

The computer is a tool; it is a means to an end. There are things that it can do as well as things that it cannot do.

Hardware

Hardware is the physical machinery, e.g. the computer itself and anything attached to it. I am not going to discuss hardware in detail. You will need a computer that has:

- A fast enough **processor** – the main computing element of the computer, the engine of the computer
- Enough **memory** – space on the computer for storing data that can be accessed quickly but is lost when the computer is switched off
- Enough **disk space** – where data are stored for later use, for example data that were in memory and now need to be kept

- **Peripherals** – items attached to the computer such as printers, scanners, CD-ROMs, etc.

- **Internet access** – to access the World Wide Web and e-mail, typically using a modem and a dial-up link.

Your supplier will be able to advise on an appropriate set-up for your needs.

I am assuming that you can use a keyboard and mouse, can copy to a disk drive, print to a printer and access the Internet to use e-mail and the World Wide Web (a massive resource, where huge amounts of information are available from the Internet). This is all you really need to be able to do to get started. There are basic computer skills courses run in your local university or college that address these basic skills. There are also excellent texts, such as Cooper 2001.

Operating systems

All computers need an operating system that performs the basic functions of the computer and allows programs to be run on it. In practice you may not care about the operating system, and many users do not even know which one they are using. The look and feel of the computer will to some extent be affected by the operating system chosen, so a Macintosh computer looks and behaves slightly differently from a Windows PC. However, you will probably be more interested in the applications (programs) that run under these operating systems.

You will probably be using a PC or a Macintosh computer. If you are using the latter you will be using one of the Macintosh operating systems. If you have a PC you may be using one of the Windows operating systems. Alternatively you may choose to use Linux, a version of the mainframe operating system UNIX that runs on PCs.

Which operating system you employ will be in part personal preference and in part dependent on the sort of work you do. Many graphic designers prefer the Macintosh, as it has particularly good facilities for this sort of work. Most business and general-purpose work is conducted on a PC under Windows. Many academics, especially in computing, engineering and pure science, like Linux. As Linux has a huge amount of *open source* software (open source is freely available and may be copied, and even adapted; it is not necessarily free, although much is available at no cost), it is increasing in popularity even among non-technical users.

Software

Software is the term for all the programs (also called applications) that run under a given operating system on the computer.

I am assuming you can use a:

- **word processor**, to create and edit text documents
- **web** browser, to access the World Wide Web
- **e-mail** application to read and send electronic mail.

These are covered in many texts, such as Cooper (2001).

Antivirus software

Computer viruses are malicious programs. They are typically spread by e-mail (opening attachments in e-mail is a particular hazard, and you should not open an attachment unless you are happy that it is free from viruses) or by using an infected disk (i.e. a disk that has a virus on it). Most of the time they are simply irritating, accessing your e-mail directory and e-mailing everyone in it with some message (although even this can be very damaging to your reputation, or embarrassing – some viruses take bits of text from your computer and send them out by e-mail) and possibly infecting their computers. Some of them are physically damaging, and you could have all your data deleted by a virus.

It is very important that you have antivirus software installed on your computer. Examples include Norton Antivirus, MacAfee Antivirus and F-Secure (on http://www. F-Secure.com or http://www. Europe. F-Secure.com). These will protect your computer against known viruses and, if you keep them updated, emerging viruses are unlikely to infect your computer either.

Databases

Creating and using databases can be necessary to you as a student if the work you are doing for your course involves listing and sorting information. If you are undertaking a research project, for example, you may wish as part of your study to ask questions and record the answers in a way that allows you to retrieve these answers at a later date. Additionally, you may wish to keep a list of names and addresses of useful contacts. You could undertake both of these tasks manually with pen and paper. However, if you are handling large amounts of information, the process of checking your information and retrieving it at a later date is lengthy, tedious and time-consuming if you do it by hand. For example, if your list of contacts contains over 100 names, think of the time it will take you to write each name (last name and first name), and additional data for each, such as address, phone number, job title, place of work, area of expertise – and to do this in alphabetical order! Obviously, you could write all this information, person by person, on individual cards and place them in a box file in alphabetical order. However, in 4 months time you may remember that one of the 100 people on your list has a particular area of expertise that you need. If you do all of this manually, you will have to read through the entire card file, name by name, to find the person who has the expertise you are seeking. Equally, you may need to categorize each of your 100 people by job title or by place of work. If you do it manually, you will need to write a whole new list or set of cards for these 100 people under the heading you want.

Database software provides a very simple solution to the above situation. A database is like an electronic filing system where any one piece of information stored acts as a basis for sorting and retrieving any information that has been stored in the database (or electronic filing system). Here is an example:

Let us go back to the list of 100 contact names that you want to keep in your filing system. For each of the 100 people you can create a database that records the following (Fig. 4.1):

- last name
- first name
- address
- post code
- telephone number

FIGURE 4.1	**Example of a record**

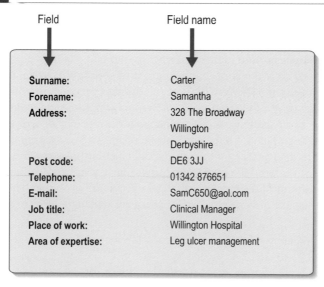

Field   Field name

Surname: Carter
Forename: Samantha
Address: 328 The Broadway
                        Willington
                        Derbyshire
Post code: DE6 3JJ
Telephone: 01342 876651
E-mail: SamC650@aol.com
Job title: Clinical Manager
Place of work: Willington Hospital
Area of expertise: Leg ulcer management

- e-mail address
- job title
- place of work
- area of expertise.

Each of these bullet points is called a field name. Next to each field name is a space (which is called the field) into which the appropriate information is entered. All the fields together make up a record, which is unique to each of the 100 people. A group of records is a file and one or more files collectively make up the database.

To summarize, think of a database as a filing cabinet. Each drawer in the filing cabinet is the same as a file. Each document in each of the suspended 'slots' in each drawer is the same as a record and each 'name tab' clipped on to the top of the suspended 'slots' in the filing cabinet drawer is the same as a field name.

Once you have created the database with all your 100 names, addresses and so forth, you can then sort and retrieve the information in any form you want using any one of the fields:

- You can call up a list of all people whose job title is 'Clinical Manager'
- You can call up a list of all people with expertise in leg ulcer management
- You can call up a list of all people who work in Willington Hospital.

Calling up a list based on a particular field is known as undertaking a search or query.

Setting up a database needs some careful thought. For example, if you think that in the future you might want to retrieve a list of all the people in your database who live in a particular county, then you need to make sure that you create a separate field called 'county'. If in the future you will want to contact everyone on your list over the age of 40, then you need to create a separate field called 'age'.

Most database software packages can print out a report for you so that you have a hard copy of the results of your search or query. Most can also perform basic statistical calculations, which is useful if you are undertaking research. However, if you are dealing with a large amount of data, especially figures, you are probably better off using a purpose-designed statistical software package, or a spreadsheet.

Spreadsheets

A spreadsheet is a particular piece of computer software that enables you to both record and process numerical information and

FIGURE 4.2	*A basic spreadsheet*

	A	B	C	D
1				
2				
3				23
4				12
5				35
6				16
7				
8				

to undertake arithmetical and statistical operations on these numerical data. The basic appearance of a spreadsheet is shown in Figure 4.2.

Each column of the spreadsheet is identified by a letter and each row by a number. The box where a column and a row meet is called a cell. Each cell has its own 'address', which is derived from the letter column and row number (e.g. A6 or B4).

If you look at Figure 4.2, what is the address of the cell that has the number 16 in it?

If you answered D6, then you are right.

Cells may contain text (titles, headings), values (numbers) or formulae (for mathematical or statistical calculations). Spreadsheets are particularly useful for formulae and it is in this area that they are far more useful than electronic calculators.

As an example, look at the four numbers in column D of Figure 4.2. You could easily add these up manually and record the sum of the four numbers in cell D7. You do not necessarily even need a calculator to do this as there are so few numbers that it is an easy task to complete manually. However, look at Figure 4.3. Here you will see a spreadsheet with a list of numbers. You could add the 16 numbers up manually – but it would take a while to do it. You could use an electronic calculator and it would do it more quickly. Or you could use the spreadsheet to add up all the numbers and record the sum of all 16 figures in cell D18.

You may ask 'Why should I use a spreadsheet to do this addition when a calculator is almost as quick?'. The answer is because a

FIGURE 4.3   *Spreadsheet with calculation*

	A	B	C	D
1				54.89
2				95.37
3				2.60
4				23.67
5				66.12
6				34.67
7				21.09
8				39.88
9				40.05
10				79.99
11				23.11
12				13.90
13				54.33
14				98.37
15				51.22
16				78.39
17				
18				777.65

spreadsheet is particularly useful when any numbers in the cells change for any reason. Unlike a calculator, where you must type in the figures individually to get the sum total (54.89 + 95.37 + 2.60 + 23.67 and so forth), with a spreadsheet you instruct the computer to add the cells together (D1 + D2 + D3 + D4 and so forth). In this way, if you later change any figures in the columns, the spreadsheet notices this and recalculates the total automatically.

Is there any way that a spreadsheet might be of use to you at work or in your studies?

Spreadsheets are typically used for things like keeping accounts, planning budgets and dealing with wages. They can also be used for planning off-duty rota sheets and are often used effectively by managers to make projections. For example, if there is a 4% rise in nursing salaries, a spreadsheet can quickly show the manager how this will affect the total salary bill.

FIGURE 4.4   *Picture of a house using tools in a word processing package*

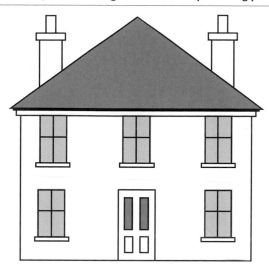

At home, you can use a spreadsheet to keep track of your bank accounts, or record the income and expenditure of a local club or organization.

Graphics and drawing

You will probably have noticed the clever use of title sequences before a television programme begins, or the cartoons and moving logos that are so eye-catching in television advertisements. These are made possible through sophisticated graphics and drawing software packages. Smaller and less expensive graphics and drawing packages are available for individuals to use on their own desktop or laptop computers. These can be used to add diagrams or pictures to your project work, reports and essays, or to produce greeting cards, posters and brochures for home or work.

The word 'graphics' refers to everything from a simple black and white drawing using shapes (Fig. 4.4) to complex colour images that can move. Most of the illustrations in this book have been produced using some sort of graphics software package.

Graphics packages come in different forms and can be used in different ways. The simple drawing in Figure 4.1 can be produced by the drawing tools that come as part of standard word processing packages. If you have time, patience and skill you can use graphics packages to produce your own pictures and diagrams from scratch, and these may be quite detailed, complex and sophisticated.

There is a graphics package called clip art that often comes as a standard part of the software provided when you buy a computer. You may also buy various clip art graphics packages, which contain hundreds of images and pictures – some in cartoon form, others not – which you can retrieve and use as they are or customize to suit your needs. They are usually free of copyright so you can use them without seeking anyone's permission.

Another alternative is to use an electronic scanner, which can be attached to your computer and allows you to reproduce a picture electronically and use it in your own report, essay or document. Care must be taken, however, not to infringe copyright law.

A useful resource is the ability to download photographs and graphics images from the Internet so that you can then include them in presentations, posters and assignments. However, there are copyright implications in doing this. Sometimes a website will say that anyone is free to use any of the material (including pictures and graphics) without seeking any further copyright clearance. Where there is no mention of this on a particular website, you are obliged under copyright law to seek clearance from the webmaster of that website to download the material on to your own computer for your use. The webmaster is the person who controls, builds and updates the website.

Digital cameras and digital video cameras are now relatively cheap, and these can be directly connected to computers, allowing pictures and video to be put on your computer. They should come with software to edit the images or film clips.

In summary, graphics and drawing packages, as well as the Internet, can be used to enhance your presentation, whether this is for an assignment, poster, seminar or group presentation as part of your studies or your work.

THE DATA PROTECTION ACT

Anyone who uses a computer to store, retrieve and use personal information about other people needs to be aware of the Data Protection Act 1998. This Act of Parliament replaced the earlier Data Protection Act 1984 and was passed to create tighter standards of practice for people and institutions that hold, in an electronic format, potentially sensitive data about people. The Data Protection Act lays down the responsibilities of those who hold the data (users) and the rights of the people on whom data are electronically held (subjects). All those who store, use and retrieve potentially sensitive data about other individuals should have a copy of the Data Protection Act. The information section at the end of this chapter will tell you how to get a copy of the Data Protection Act 1998.

The Act indicates that all data users must register with the Data Protection Register and must comply with the principles of data protection as laid down in the Act. A summary of these principles is given in Box 4.1.

BOX 4.1	**Summary of the principles of the Data Protection Act**
	Personal data should be:

Personal data should be:
- Collected and processed fairly and lawfully
- Held and used only for specified and lawful purposes
- Adequate, relevant and accurate
- Held for no longer than is necessary for the registered purpose
- Protected by proper security.

Failure to comply with the provisions of the Act can lead to prosecution. You can receive a copy of an information pack on the Data Protection Act specifically designed for students by contacting the address at the end of this chapter.

SEARCHING THE INTERNET

How can you access information on the Internet for your studies?

The first thing you need to do is to gain access to the Internet. If you are studying at a university, this will be possible through the computers in your university. Increasingly, hospitals and health practices have computers with Internet access.

If you have your own computer at home, you will be able to get Internet access from a huge number of companies (including Orange, Sky, Microsoft, Virgin, AOL, BT and even WH Smith and Tesco). Most of us are constantly reminded of this with free offers of Internet access coming through the post, on television and on advertising hoardings. It is important when subscribing to an Internet provider that you take into account the cost of telephone calls because each time you access a website it amounts to the cost of a local telephone call. Many telephone providers have special offers that reduce your telephone call charges at certain times when you use the Internet. Increasingly, broadband is available, which is much faster but also more expensive. Access via cable may be available to you, depending where you live, and you may also be able to access the Internet via a wireless connection. If you are an occasional user of the Internet, dial-up on an ordinary phone line with a modem is acceptable. If you use the Internet a lot (daily for more than half an hour) or if you need to download large files a lot, broadband may be a viable alternative. Broadband costs about £20–30 per month, but there are typically no extra charges however long you are on the Internet, and you have a telephone line as well as one for the Internet.

If you are a personal subscriber to an Internet provider, the instructions for how to access the Internet will be given to you when you subscribe to that Internet provider. In a university, Internet access is through the university's Internet server, and all networked computers should have access to the Internet at all times.

All websites on the computer have a dedicated 'address' called a URL (uniform resource locator). If you know the URL of a particular site, all you need to do to access the site is to access your Internet server's website and then, where you see the box labelled 'Address' at the top of your Internet server's home page, type in the URL and press the 'return' key on your keyboard. Depending on the speed of your server's link, you will quickly see the home page of your selected website come up on the screen. You then follow the instructions on the home page to access other pages on that website. This usually is through 'clicking' (using the left-hand button on your mouse) on to a word or picture with your mouse or through typing in some words in a particular box and then pressing the 'return' key.

If you have access to a computer with Internet access, try the following:

1. Access the home page of the Internet server. This may happen automatically when you turn the computer on. Alternatively, there may be an icon (symbol) on your screen that you can 'click' on to get into the Internet.
2. In the 'Address' box, type in the following URL: http://www.ask.co.uk
3. This will take you to a website called 'Ask Jeeves'. The website asks you to type in a question.
4. In the 'Question' box, either type your own question to ask Jeeves or else type in 'Where can I find a map of London?'
5. When you have typed your question, click on the word 'Ask' next to the question box.
6. What have you found?

You have just used one of the many search engines for the Internet.

What does a search engine allow you to do?

Search engines allow you to find things on the Internet. You type in key words related to the information you would like to find and a search engine will give you a list of the websites where you can find the information you are seeking. The activity you did (above) is an example of one search engine called 'Ask Jeeves'.

There are many search engines available; each is located at a different website. Some search engines are US-based while others are

TABLE 4.1	*Examples of search engines*
Name of search engine	**Web address (URL)**
Google	http://www.google.co.uk
Yahoo	http://www.yahoo.com
Lycos	http://www.lycos.co.uk
Excite	http://www.excite.com
MSN	http://www.msn.co.uk
Alta Vista	http://jump.altavista.com
Ask Jeeves	http://www.ask.co.uk

UK-based. Some of the most common search engines are listed in Table 4.1.

Although these websites may look quite different from each other, they all work in almost the same way. Towards the top of each of these search engine web pages will be a box that says SEARCH. You will be able to type a key word or phrase in that box. If you type a phrase (rather than an individual word) in the search box, it is helpful to type it in double quotation marks (" ") to avoid the search engine finding information about the separate words rather than the phrase (i.e. if you want to search for information on health education, type it as "health education").

Next to the search box where you have typed in your key words is a button which says 'Go' or 'Search' or 'Go get it'. Click on this button using the left-hand button on your mouse. This tells the search engine to find the information you are seeking.

What will come up on your screen is a list of websites related to the key words you typed in the search box. Using the mouse, you can click on any of these websites and immediately go to that site to get the information you need. Not all websites will automatically have what you are looking for but this will depend on the nature of the search and how specific you were when typing in your key words. General, broad key words will give you hundred or thousands of websites that will prove to be of little or no use to you. Very specific search instructions will probably provide you with information you really can use.

Alternatively, instead of using a search engine you could access a directory, where information is stored in a structured format on a given subject. For nursing, midwifery and allied health there is, for example, nmap.ac.uk, which offers useful links. An example of links found for pressure ulcer is shown in Figure 4.5, compared with a search conducted on Google (www.google.co.uk).

FIGURE 4.5   *Links found for pressure ulcer on (a) NMAP (b) Google*

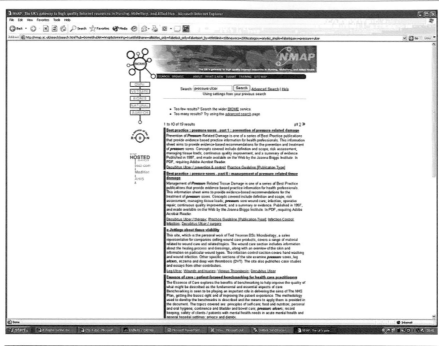

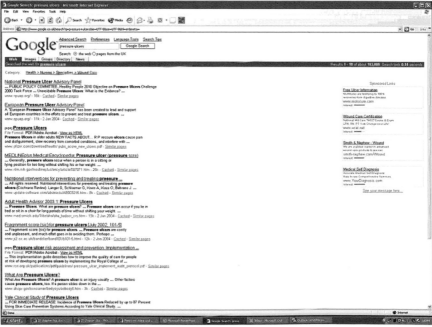

How do I know if the information I find on a website is accurate and valid?

The Internet is a free place and, provided you know how to set up your own web page, you can publish anything on the Internet with little or no academic scrutiny or critical review. There is an extremely wide variety of information available on the Internet with varying degrees of accuracy, reliability and value. No one has to approve the content before it goes on the Internet. Therefore, it is up to individual users to critically evaluate Internet sources of information and research. Harris has posted a guide for evaluating the quality of Internet sources on to the Internet and it is essential for all students to become familiar with this skill.

Harris identifies several things that need to be looked at to evaluate sources from the Internet:

■ **Screening information:** matching a site with what you are looking for; looking for papers that are factual and well argued with supported claims, considering whether you have enough information about the source of the website to feel that the material might be reliable and accurate

■ **Tests of information quality:** Harris offers the CARS checklist for information quality – Credibility, Accuracy, Reasonableness and Support. Each of these is comprehensively explained on Harris's website, which is http://www.sccu.edu/faculty/RHarris/evalu8it.htm.

One problem that has worsened with the Internet is plagiarism. It is possible to download material from the Internet and pass it off as your own. This is considered to be an academic offence in all universities, and proven plagiarism will normally lead to disciplinary action. If you always reference any material that is not your own, and make it clear when you are quoting from another work, you should have no problems.

CLINICAL PROBLEM

For the remainder of this chapter I will consider a clinical problem, and see how IT can help to solve it. Applications shown in these sections are important if you want to conduct research and may be useful if you have to write a dissertation for your study.

The problem to be investigated is the importance of different risk factors for the development of pressure ulcers in immobilized patients. Only certain components of the Waterlow score (Waterlow 1985) were relevant in each clinical area (Anthony *et al.*, 1998, 2000a), but different components in different areas. (The Waterlow score consists of eleven subscores, including gender, age, mobility, continence, recent surgery and other special risks, and other factors thought to be relevant in pressure sore incidence.) Also, it has been shown beyond reasonable doubt that serum albumin (a measure of nutrition) is relevant over and above the Waterlow score in predicting those patents who are at risk of pressure ulcers (Anthony *et al.*, 2000b).

But what does this mean in practice, i.e. how does this impact on the care of a patient. In principle if we know who is at most risk, we should be able to allocate resources to those patients to reduce that risk (e.g. pressure-relieving devices) but there is little evidence that this in fact is the case.

If you were to deal with the issue, you would want to assess the impact of reduction of pressure ulcers, and it would be helpful to first assess what happens to a patient who has one, compared to one who does not.

Consider what different outcomes two patients may have. One has a pressure ulcer, one does not.

Many different outcomes may be seen in the two patients. The pressure ulcer patient may develop infection at the wound site, may suffer pain, may feel depressed about the ulcer or embarrassed by the smell of the wound. One major impact may be that it is difficult to discharge the patient, and s/he may stay in hospital longer.

Using the Internet to conduct a literature review

Let us explore the problem of increased length of stay in hospital (LOS), as this is important to the patient, who probably wants to go home, and to the hospital, which wants the bed to treat more patients. First we need to find out what is known about pressure ulcers and LOS. We need to conduct a review of the literature. Increasingly we are asked to conduct reviews systematically. A systematic review is one where we are precise about how we conduct the review, and state how we have performed it such that another person using the information we record would come up with an identical set of papers and a similar view of the literature.

How would you plan such a review? Where would you search for this information, from what date would you want to explore the literature, in which languages, in which type of journal, what type of study, using what types of database? You might look at http://www.york.ac.uk/dept/crd or http://www.nelh.ac.uk for ideas.

You would probably look in medical, nursing and allied health bibliographic databases as the subject is clinical, such as MEDLINE and CINAHL. Since pressure ulcer research is not as time-sensitive as (say) policy issues or technological innovations, you would probably search from the start of the databases, which is from the 1960s for MEDLINE and the 1980s for CINAHL. You would be most interested in empirical studies with data on LOS, using an appropriate methodology. You might also explore Cochrane (accessible via http://www.nelh.nhs.uk) for systematic reviews. You might hand-search (i.e. look through every issue) of relevant specialist journals such as the *Journal of Wound Care*. You would probably restrict yourself to one or a few languages (although most articles indexed in MEDLINE and CINAHL are in English).

You could use a CD-ROM in the library but it is probably easier to use the Internet to access the bibliographic databases. For example you could go to http://www.library.dmu.ac.uk and click on 'databases' and then select the databases you wish to access – ones to do with health, possibly MEDLINE or CINAHL.

For example, a year ago I searched MEDLINE for medical subheadings (MESH) keywords 'length of stay' AND 'pressure ulcer'. A total of 91 articles were returned, the date range being 1971–2002.

In addition to the bibliographic database search, you should consider using the Web as a resource. Employing a search engine (see above) you may find further information that is not published (possibly in researchers' own web home pages), or not found in my previous search.

What problems might there be with information found on the Web? What quality assurance criteria might you employ to check the validity of these pages?

In many, although not all, cases, material on the Internet has not been subject to peer review scrutiny, and there may be bias. The authority of the author may be questionable; the information may be purely marketing material. However if you employ a good checklist you should still be able to use web-based material. There are many such checklists available in textbooks or on the Web, or you could use the CARS checklist discussed earlier in this chapter. Essentially you want to consider the authority of the authors (are they competent, qualified, attached to a respected institution, etc.?), the timeliness (is it recent?), the level (do you understand it, is it too basic?) and the relevance.

In many cases the papers are available in full text, typically in portable document format (PDF), which you will probably not be able to view on your word processor. You need a separate, but free, package called Adobe Acrobat Reader, which you can download from http://www.acrobat.com. There is a more complete version of Adobe Acrobat, with added features, for which payment is required, but you probably only need the simple free program. PDF files show you the paper exactly as in the printed page of the journal, which is why they are used often in preference to (say) web files (HTML), which differ depending on your screen size, resolution and how your computer is set up. PDF files have a major advantage in that, if you refer to a page or set of pages, any reader will be able to access the correct pages.

Some articles I located were worth getting in full. These are the articles that appear to be relevant, based on the titles, keywords and, where available, the abstract. I could in many cases get these from my library, which is about 50 yards from my office in the university. This is not going to be convenient to most clinicians, and is only of use to me if the article is in the library. An alternative is to use the Internet to download the text, which may be free, if my institution subscribes to the text, or I may need to pay for it. Rather than access the site of the journal, I prefer to use the Athens system. The advantage is that, instead of having to register and use a different password for each journal, Athens give you one user-code and password, and all journals signing up to Athens (a very big proportion of the ones I care about) are available in full text. I tend to go to the Ingenta system to get full text, which is obtainable from the Bath Information Data Service (BIDS) at http://www.bids.ac.uk.

I can now go through the references, which include the abstracts. What I discover is that there is a lot of material suggesting that pressure ulcers and LOS are related, and that patients with pressure ulcers have greater LOS.

Can you describe the typical patient with pressure ulcers? How might they be different from patients without pressure ulcers? Does this have any bearing on LOS?

They may be older and are more likely to be incontinent, diabetic, confused, immobile, smokers, have had recent surgery or trauma, or have higher scores on any of the Waterlow subscores. As they are more ill, they may stay in hospital longer because of their greater morbidity rather than because they have pressure ulcers.

Reference management

Having done my review I needed to store my references so that when I later write a paper or report I can refer to them.

How would you store these references?

You could take hard copies of any full papers you photocopied, or downloaded over the Internet, and put them in a folder, in a box or on a shelf for later use. You could take the details of each paper and put them in a card index box, or listed on paper, stored in a word processor document, or on a database such as Access. However there is a better way – use a reference management system, which is a database specifically designed to store bibliographic references.

Reference management systems have been available for many years. A reference management system allows you to store references in a database and insert them as needed as citations into an essay, paper, thesis or other document. The program typically operates from within your selected word processor, and can automatically produce the correct format of citation and the appropriate reference list. You can change the output reference list and the citations referring to it by directing the program via a simple 'switch' to, say, use the Vancouver or the Harvard system.

This is useful for a variety of reasons. It is simple, it is efficient, you can use the same references in more than one document with no extra typing, the reference list is always complete, and all citations refer to a reference and all references have a citation. This is particularly useful in long documents.

Early reference management systems included Refer and BibTeX, originally designed for the UNIX operating system. An early reference management system operating on DOS (a basic operating system used on PCs before Windows) was Papyrus. However these systems are not as easy to use as the more recent Windows-based systems. There are many reference management systems that run on PCs and on Macintosh computers; examples include Procite, Reference Manager and EndNote. These systems are all functionally similar, and probably all the modern systems do much the same thing. The use of EndNote within Microsoft Word is shown in Figure 4.6. EndNote and some other reference management software, when it is installed, creates a new item in the Tools menu in Microsoft Word (for example) and from within Word I can ask for a reference that is already created in EndNote. Some reference management software (EndNote and Reference Manager for example) allow you to directly import references from bibliographic databases, so you do not even need to type them in once.

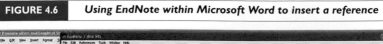

FIGURE 4.6   *Using EndNote within Microsoft Word to insert a reference*

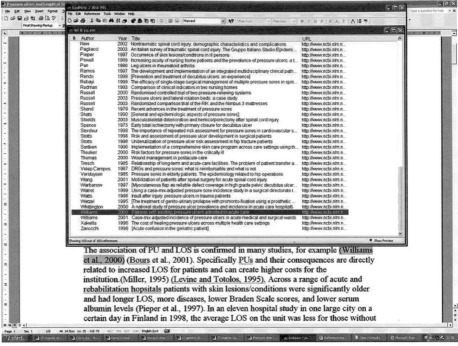

Hospital information support systems

From my literature review I am not sure whether LOS is caused by pressure ulcers or merely associated with it, as patients with pressure ulcers are in any event much more ill and frail. My colleagues in Burton have a Hospital Information Support System (HISS) on which is recorded patient data. This is a computerized system.

Hospital Information Support Systems are databases, although very large and complicated ones. Clinical data are stored on a HISS, and may include medical notes, nursing notes, laboratory data and other patient data.

The great advantage of HISSs is that authorized users can access data as soon as it is entered on the system. Furthermore, multiple copies can be read, so more than one health professional can see the data at the same time. For example, both the ward manager and the doctor can access the laboratory results on the same patient simultaneously. HISSs or similar systems can be the basis for an electronic patient record (EPR). The aim of an EPR is to allow all health professionals to be able to access relevant data at any time and from any location. The EPR can automatically follow the patient, as it will still be available if the patient is transferred and should be immediately available when the patient is admitted. The doctor cannot take the patient notes off the ward, and there should never be missing notes.

While the HISS is typically used to treat patients, here I want to use it for audit or research.

Statistical packages

I use the Statistical Package for Social Sciences (SPSS) and want to analyse these data. SPSS is like a specialized spreadsheet with additional statistical, graphical and reporting facilities. SPSS is a complex package but there are many texts discussing its use; for example, one I like is by Bryman and Cramer (1999), and for nurse researchers there is Anthony (1999).

SPSS is useful for small datasets. For example, if you have data on even a few dozen patients it is easier to use SPSS than to conduct the analysis manually. Burton had data on hundreds of thousands of patients, and using a statistics package is the only practical way to conduct the analysis. Also, once data are entered, I can produce tables, plot graphs and conduct statistical tests very easily. Some differences between manual statistical analysis and the use of a package are shown in Table 4.2.

It would be great to download the data straight into SPSS. This is probably possible, but I know it is possible to download the data from the proprietary software to an Access database, which is an industry standard. SPSS did not at the time support Access, but Access can export data into the Microsoft Excel spreadsheet, and SPSS can read Excel files. The upshot is, with a bit of fiddling, I can download patients' data into my chosen statistics package. I have of course, prior to this applied to the relevant ethics committees and obtained permission to use their data, and I have had the data anonymized (see earlier section on data protection) prior to receiving it, so no patient is identifiable.

In this section I am using a graph called a boxplot. It is not necessary here to fully understand the boxplot, what is important is that it gives useful information on groups of patients. First I perform a boxplot of those patients with pressure ulcers against those with none. A boxplot show you a lot of information on some variable, such as LOS in days (Fig. 4.7). The range of values from lowest to highest is shown as two short horizontal lines. In practice extreme values (outliers) are removed, so we see the range of the overwhelming majority of the data, missing possibly a few really odd values. Between these high and low points is a vertical line with a box in it. This box contains half the data. Within the box is a straight line, which marks the median value.

TABLE 4.2	Statistics conducted manually versus using statistical software	
	Manual (pen and paper) statistics	**Statistical software**
Inputting data	You will want to have data in an optimal form for conducting analysis. This may mean having several forms of the data on paper	Input data once
Statistical formulae	You will need to know these and be able to manipulate them	You only need to know the test you want to conduct, not how to compute it
Errors in calculation	You may not know you have made an error, and if you do you will need to recalculate	The software should not make errors of this type
New data, or input data corrected	You will need to recalculate	The computer will recalculate when you ask for the analysis again. You can save analyses into a special file and simply call it up
Inappropriate test used	You can use the wrong test but if you know statistics well enough to compute manually, it is likely you will know when to use a given test	You can ask the computer to conduct almost any test on almost any data. The software is in general not able to detect that you are doing the wrong thing
Many different statistical approaches needed on data	You will need to recalculate for each test, or plot each graph or produce each table individually	You can ask the software to conduct many tests, plot graphs and produce tables once the data are input

FIGURE 4.7	Boxplot showing the effect of pressure ulcers on length of stay in hospital

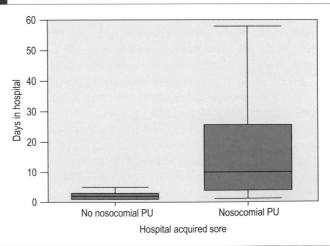

So a lot of information is seen in a boxplot. Here we can see that the patients with pressure ulcers have in general a much greater LOS. The range for pressure ulcer patients shows that the bottom and top values for LOS are higher, as the nosocomial (i.e. occurred in hospital) pressure ulcer has a range of about 1–58 days, compared with about 1–5 days for those with no ulcer. Also, the box showing where 50% of the patients lie is much higher, and the median is higher. So all three measures show that pressure ulcer patients have greater LOS.

However we know that there may be confounding factors. For example, the various risk factors of the Waterlow score could mostly be associated with greater LOS. What if I were to try to allow for these by taking only patients in a given risk group, say only those with a high risk? Then if it were the risk factors rather than the pressure ulcers that were causing greater LOS the plots should be similar. In fact when I selected only those patients with the same Waterlow score, there was still a greater LOS associated with the pressure ulcer group. It looks as if pressure ulcers may cause greater LOS rather than just being associated with it.

Presentation software

Suppose that, having explored pressure ulcers and LOS, you decide that we need to get the hospital trust to support further work. It would be useful to get the chief executive of the trust on board. You may need to do a presentation, and here presentation software will help. You may later want to give a lecture at a conference, or give a teaching session. All of these could be helped using such presentation software. You could use Microsoft PowerPoint, but there are other packages, including those running on Linux (an alternative operating system to Windows), that are functionally similar.

I have taken some graphical output from SPSS and copied it directly to PowerPoint. There are several ways to do this, but one very simple way is to use the 'Edit' then 'Copy' pull-down menu in SPSS (and most other Windows packages, such as Word and PowerPoint) from within SPSS. This copies the graph into the Windows clipboard (an area copied to and from Windows programs). In PowerPoint I can do 'Edit' then 'Paste' and the graphic will appear in my PowerPoint presentation (Fig. 4.8). I could also have done this to include the boxplot in a Word document, for example an academic paper I intended to send to a journal.

Qualitative analysis packages

Thus far we have assumed that our data are quantitative, and have employed SPSS for the analysis. However, suppose that, instead of

| FIGURE 4.8 | *Using Microsoft PowerPoint* |

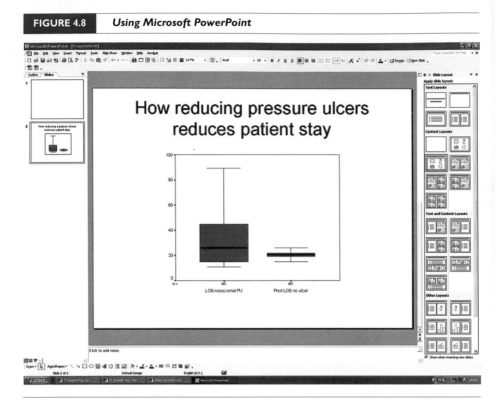

taking numerical data about patients, I interviewed them. Let us assume that I want to know what it is like to have a pressure ulcer. I have a set of questions I want to ask, possibly asking patients to rank their pain on a 1–10 scale, for example. This is clearly quantitative data (although based on subjective assessment). However I may also ask them to put in their own words how they feel. What I get back will not be analysable with a statistics package like SPSS. There are a whole range of qualitative packages. If you access one of the web pages for qualitative analysis, such as http://www.car.ua.edu/ or http://www.umich.edu/~qualnet/resources.htm, you will see a list of them.

Just because the technology exists, it is not necessary to use it. You can perform qualitative analysis manually. However if you are going to do a lot of qualitative analysis, or will be working in a team, it may be of advantage to learn to use a qualitative analysis package. For a discussion of the advantages and disadvantages of qualitative data analysis software, see Lee and Esterhuizen (2000) or Maclaran and Catterall (2002).

You can download a demonstration package of one of the market leaders, NVivo, from http://www.qsr.com.au/. There are also free packages from the Centers for Disease Control and Prevention in the USA. AnSWR is on http://www.cdc.gov/nchstp/hiv_aids/software/answr.htm and CDC EZ-Text is on http://www.cdc.gov/nchstp/hiv_aids/software/ez-text.htm.

Clinical guidelines

By now I think I know that pressure ulcers are a big problem, I would like to institute some intervention that reduces the incidence of pressure ulcers. What I need is a clinical guideline. A clinical guideline is the result of a systematic review that is used to inform clinical practice by creating an evidence-based document.

Consider a nurse on a medical ward, who may need to have the most up-to-date practice for diabetes, heart disease, rheumatoid arthritis and many other diseases. All nurses should base their practice on research but no clinical nurse has the time to personally review the academic press on any given subject, let alone all the areas they may need to address.

Clinical guidelines are produced by teams of experts to deal with specific conditions. Increasingly, these are available on the Internet – for example the National Electronic Library for Health (UK) on http://www.nelh.nhs.uk, the National Guideline Clearing House (USA) on http://www.guideline.gov and, my personal favourite, the Scottish Intercollegiate Guidelines Network on http://www.sign.ac.uk are all sites that offer clinical guidelines.

Suppose you want to reduce the incidence of pressure ulcers. If a clinical guideline exists that would help to reduce pressure ulcers then I could use this in an audit programme. Indeed, on searching via the National Electronic Library for Health on http://www.nelh.nhs.uk, which has a clinical guideline finder, I can find a clinical guideline for pressure ulcer prevention (Fig. 4.9).

Web page design

Suppose you have now written a paper based on my work on pressure ulcers and LOS. At this point you want to add the paper to your curriculum vitae (CV). It is common practice for academics to do this, as others may want to know, for example, the type of work a given academic or team is involved in. If I come across a paper that is of interest, I may access the personal web page of the author to see what else they have published, or even not yet published. My CV is on the web – you can see it at http://www.dmu.ac.uk/~danthony (Fig. 4.10). How do I do this?

There are several ways. You might use a specialist web authoring program, such as Microsoft FrontPage, although there are many

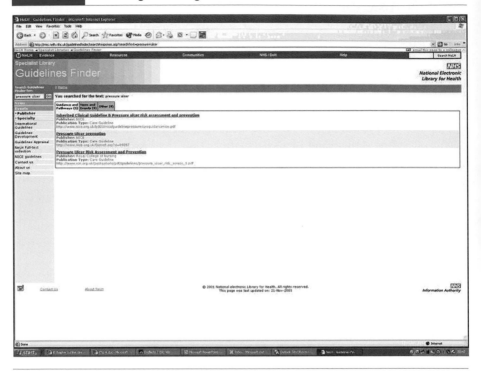

FIGURE 4.9   *Locating a clinical guideline*

other such packages, some of them freely available on the Web, some free, and many available on the Linux system. Using such a package you can create hyperlinked documents fairly easily and, if you have your own webspace via your organization or your Internet provider (these days most will give you some space, many of them at no extra cost, which you can access with a user-code and password), you can upload the document. This is called publishing the document in FrontPage, and is a simple process, involving putting in the user-code and password for your webspace. Once uploaded, the file can potentially be viewed by anyone with a web browser, i.e. virtually anyone at all. They will need to know what the file is called, or much more probably you will have linked the document into a special page called the home page, which is the one all users access automatically when they access your site.

So on my site, there is a home page. Note that I have downloaded a picture of myself taken with a digital camera and copied directly onto my PC (I could have scanned a normal photo). On my home page I have linked the CV. Clicking on the CV will show you the file with the added paper. (Currently this is not published, and I have put it in

FIGURE 4.10   *My web page*

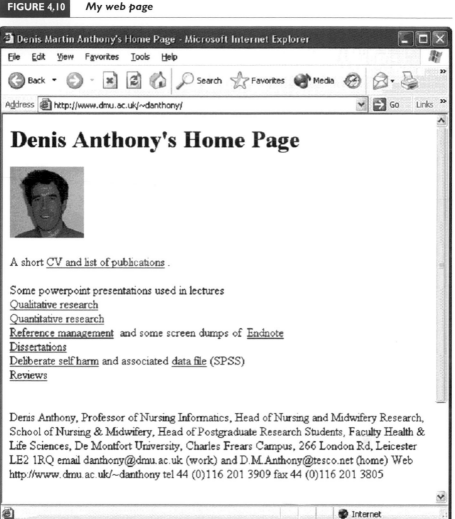

the papers in preparation section. If it gets published I will move it into the main section.)

Web authoring packages can be complicated, not very easy to use, not robust and with many features in which you are not interested. I often want to update a page when I do not have the software with me (I travel and use Internet cafes a lot). You may not wish to purchase further software (although increasingly FrontPage comes as a standard on new PCs). You can edit web pages perfectly adequately in Word or other word processing packages. Some complex pages are difficult to

| FIGURE 4.11 | *Using an FTP program to transfer a file to a website* |

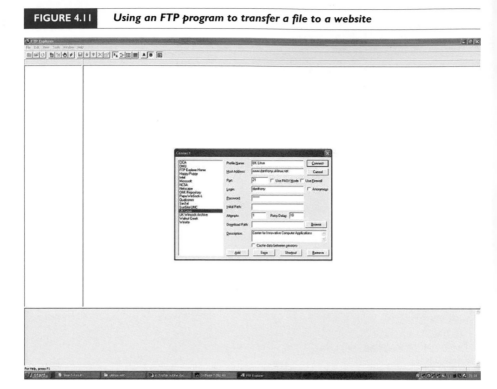

edit in Word, as it is not designed for web page editing, and there are some strange behaviours, but Word does support basic web page edit ing. Word, and other packages, even create a link for you if you enter what appears to be a web page or e-mail address. Thus when readers browse your page and see the address, they may click on it and automatically (if connected to the Internet) access that page. So I could have made my changes to the file in Word. Also if I had a pre-existing Word file (if, say, my CV was in a Word document) I could save it as a web file, using 'file' and 'save as' options in Word and choose to save as a web file. Thus I have avoided the necessity to learn any HTML (the language used to create web pages).

But how do I transfer the file?

As described above, you could have a specialized web authoring system that will do this for you. Alternatively, most computers have a file transfer protocol (ftp) program. Some of these are Windows-based, but at the very least you should be able to use a DOS-based one, which should be installed on most or all PCs, called simply ftp. You can also find ftp packages via the Web, freely available, and some are free (Fig. 4.11). In this figure I am using FTP Explorer, available on ftpx.com.

FIGURE 4.11   *(continued)*

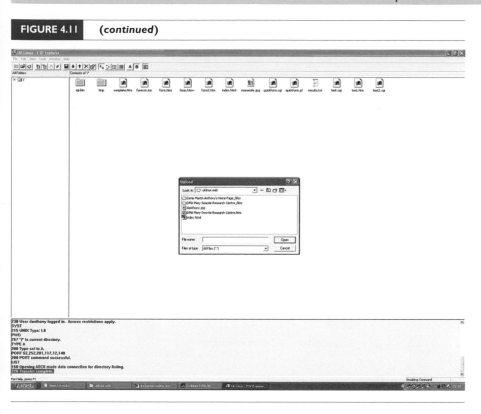

The ftp allows you to copy files from one computer to another. Here I have used it to copy a revised version of my home page (index.html) to my website. In the first screen you can see that I am connecting to one of several ftp sites, in this case my own personal site on http://www.danthony.uklinux.net, which requires me to give a user-code and a password. Once connected, the second screen is shown, which now allows me to upload files on to the site. The files already on the site are shown in the right hand side of the screen. I am copying from a part of my hard disk, and this is shown in the pop-up dialogue box in the middle of the screen.

Online courses

Finally, an outcome of the web is increased interest in online courses (Anthony 2000, 2001, 2003). These use the power of the Internet to allow distance learners to access material. However the added benefit of using web-based material is that the look and feel are familiar to anyone who is familiar with web pages.

FIGURE 4.12   *An online course for tissue viability*

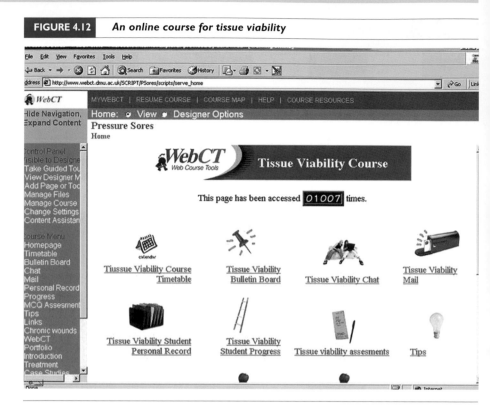

There are several virtual learning environments (VLEs) that increasingly are using web-based technology. Two common market leaders are WebCT and Blackboard, which are functionally similar. A course I used in 2000 is illustrated in Figure 4.12. This shows a menu and icons that represent various parts of the course. For example, there is a discussion board and e-mail facilities where students may talk to each other or engage in seminars. Figure 4.13 shows one of the content pages, which has many links, which will take you directly to the web page if you click on it.

The use of such a course could help keep ward staff updated on pressure ulcer treatment and prevention, to assist in the project to reduce LOS by reducing pressure ulcers incidence.

CONCLUSION

In this chapter some basic IT facilities have been outlined – hardware, software, antivirus software, databases, spreadsheets, graphics, the Data Protection Act and searching on the Internet.

FIGURE 4.13

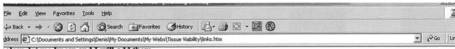

File Edit View Favorites Tools Help

← Back → · ⊗ ⌂ ⌂ ⌕Search ⌂Favorites ⌂History ⌂· ⌂ ⌂ · ⌂ ⌂

Address ⌂ C:\Documents and Settings\Denis\My Documents\My Webs\Tissue Viability\links.htm   ▾ ∂Go Link

)elow, let me know and I will add them.

General

- World Wide Wounds http://www.smtl.co.uk/World-Wide-Wounds/Common/Links.html
- OMNI on http://omni.ac.uk/umls/detail/C0011127.html is a generic health site, but has items on Decubitus Ulcer. http://members.aol.com/woundnet
- Pressure Sore Web Forum http://www.medicaledu.com/pressure_sore_forum/
- Venous Stasis Ulcer Web Forum http://www.medicaledu.com/venous_stasis_forum/
- Wound and Skin Care Links http://members.tripod.com/~DianneBrownson/wound_skin.html Dianne Brownson's 'wound and skin' links - other health care links too.
- Wound Care Information Network http://www.medicaledu.com/
- Wound Care Web Forum http://medicaledu.com/wound_care_forum/
- The Spanish nursing site http://www.readysoft.es/gneaupp/ (which has an English section on http://www.readysoft.es/gneaupp/english/index.htm).

Guidelines

- Some detailed material can be downloaded "Pressure Ulcers in Adults: Prediction and Prevention: Clinical Practice Guideline Number 3"*AHCPR Pub. No. 92-0047: May 1992* http://text.nlm.nih.gov/ftrs/tocview.
- The NHS Centre for Reviews and Dissemination at York, in particular look at http://www.york.ac.uk/inst/crd/ehc21.htm
- Scottish Intercollegiate Guidelines Network (SIGN) guidelines located at http://www.show.scot.nhs.uk/sign/
- RCN guidelines at http://www.rcn.org.uk/servicecs/promote/clinical/clinical_guidelines.htm
- Clearing House of guidelines at http://www.guidelines.gov/index.asp

http://www.medicaledu.com/pressure_sore_forum/   ⌂ My Computer

Some applications are then demonstrated with the aid of a clinical problem: pressure ulcers. After a literature review, conducted over the Internet, and some papers downloaded over the Internet, the relevant references were downloaded into a specialized database, a reference management system. A clinical guideline that would be useful was also downloaded from a specialist site. Finally, online courses were introduced that could improve patient care by educating health-care staff.

CHAPTER RESOURCES

REFERENCES

Anthony D 1999 Understanding advanced statistics: a guide for nurses and health care researchers. Churchill Livingstone, Edinburgh

Anthony D 2000 Distance learning and research dissemination using online resources. Nurse Researcher 8: 53–64

Anthony D 2001 Online course survey – some qualitative results. ITIN 13: 4–9
Anthony D 2003 Online courses in nursing and midwifery: comparisons with allied healthcare professions. British Journal of Healthcare Computing and Information Management 20: 28–30
Anthony D, Barnes J, Unsworth J 1998 An evaluation of current risk assessment scales for decubitus ulcer in general inpatients and wheelchair users. Clinical Rehabilitation 12: 136–142
Anthony D, Clark M, Dallender J 2000a An optimization of the Waterlow score using regression and artificial neural networks. Clinical Rehabilitation 14: 102–109
Anthony D, Reynolds T, Russell L 2000b An investigation into the use of serum albumin in pressure sore prediction. Journal of Advanced Nursing 32: 359–365
Bryman A, Cramer D 1999 Quantitative data analysis with SPSS Release 10 for Windows: a guide for social scientists. Routledge, Hove
Cooper C 2001 Making IT work: the Internet and IT for busy students. UWIC Press, Cardiff
Lee R, Esterhuizen L 2000 Computer software and qualitative analysis: trends, issues and resources. International Journal of Social Research Methodology 3: 231–243
Maclaran P, Catterall M 2002 Analysing qualitative data: computer software and the market research practitioner. Qualitative Market Research 5: 28–39
Waterlow J 1985 Pressure sores: a risk assessment card. Nursing Times 81(48): 49–55

5 Getting the most from reading and lectures

Kym Martindale

KEY ISSUES

- **A critical approach**
- **Reading skills**
- **Reviewing and recording**

- **The role of the lecture**
- **Note taking**
- **Engaging with the material**

INTRODUCTION

Understanding information demands effort from you, the reader/listener. Your role is not passive: for example, good note-taking skills make all the difference in the ultimate value of any material to you. Nor is your role confined simply to the time spent in the lecture or reading an article, although both these activities are part of the process of involving yourself in your learning. This process is greatly helped by you knowing what you want. As in Chapter 3, the rule is 'define and stick to your purpose'.

A CRITICAL APPROACH: SUBJECTIVITY AND INTERPRETATION

Employing a critical approach means first of all recognizing that all information is presented in an edited form. No matter what the medium – an article or book, a television or radio broadcast, or material on the Internet – the contents and presentation are chosen by authors, editors, producers, website designers and others. Such selectivity is not meant to be cunning. More often it is a response to the constraints any medium imposes, and the understanding that any material needs to be shaped for the reader/listener.

However, this does mean that those presenting and editing material do so from within their own frame of reference (Giroux 1978, cited in Baron and Sternberg 1987). A frame of reference is an individual's beliefs and values, and the factors that go towards forming them. It is unique to that person, although it is probably similar to those of other individuals. It can change but, as a teacher cited by Baron and Sternberg (1987 p. 113) states, 'at any one time, it still functions as a finite lens through which some experiences are filtered and beyond the bounds of which other experiences simply do not register'.

Two obvious examples of frame of reference influencing information are politics and newspapers. You are aware of the values and beliefs through which that speaker or journalist operates so you listen/read in a questioning light. But politicians and newspapers hold stated positions (officially or not). Most authors and contributors of Internet material are first and foremost professionals in their field. They operate through a complex system of values, beliefs, ethical concerns and cultural influences, which are not easy to detect or define. Combined with the air of authority that the media (especially print) seem to bestow, they can lull you into a false sense of acceptance.

BOX 5.1	*The great Eskimo vocabulary hoax*

A wonderful example of how print can establish error as fact is related by Stephen Pinker in *The Language Instinct*. The great Eskimo vocabulary hoax, i.e. the claim that Inuit peoples have dozens, even hundreds, of words for snow, has been widely propagated in print. The claim, originally a modest if inaccurate seven, was published in an article early in the 20th century. Successive publications inflated the claim and, with each publication, cemented the error.

Only recently have linguists returned to question the source, i.e. the original author's frame of reference and credentials.

An 'amateur scholar of Native American languages' with 'leanings towards mysticism' (Pinker 1994, p. 63), Benjamin Lee Whorf's theories were based on shaky research and clumsy translations. But the great Eskimo vocabulary hoax was compounded by a 'patronizing willingness to treat other cultures' psychologies as weird and exotic compared to our own' (Pinker 1994, p. 65). In other words, social attitudes allowed Whorf's theory to flourish without question.

How do you know who to believe?

Approaching material critically recognizes that 'I am right, they're wrong' won't always be the case. A critical approach involves you asking 'What made them reach that conclusion when they decided this?' The subject may have been differently researched, differently experienced and differently interpreted.

In considering material you have to weigh these factors and how they could affect the information you're given. You are questioning the author/editor/producer, bringing their possible frame of reference to the fore – if you can. In Chapters 8 and 9, deciding which material might be of use to you involves examining the author's credentials. This is a similar approach, but in greater depth.

Your questions won't all have answers

It is important to realize that your questions won't all have answers as such. You might not be able to find out everything you'd like to know about a piece of research or an editor's influences. You won't even always know if you have found out everything. Finally, in some cases you will have to argue that there is no hard 'yes' or 'no' answer. But the questioning is the critical and important act. It shows that you can look beyond texts and lectures.

So, you won't always know who to believe. You must appraise the evidence, both stated and implicit, and either decide for yourself or present a well-researched and clear argument as to why you cannot decide.

- Being a critical and active learner involves questioning:
  - Who is giving you your information?
  - What is their purpose and agenda?
  - What are their sources and methods of research?

- Our individual frame of reference influences our work. Objectivity is only an attempt to be disinterested; it is never possible to be utterly neutral. Remember, you too work within a frame of reference

- You won't always be able to provide answers to questions you raise, but raising them demonstrates that you have thought around the subject.

BOX 5.2	*Question . . . Concentrate . . . Understand*
	We have spent several pages addressing this issue, but it is important preparation. A questioning reader/listener is thinking and concentrating on the material. It follows that such a student stands a better chance of understanding and, in the long run, remembering.

READING: BEING PRACTICAL, REALISTIC AND PREPARED

This section will look at how reading skills vary depending on the material and your need, at how to be selective and at how to ensure you focus on your information need while reading.

Different skills for different material

You already have sophisticated reading skills and apply them every day to the various types of material you encounter. Table 5.1 lists

TABLE 5.1	*Material types and skills involved in reading different material*	
Type of material	**Purpose**	**Reading skill**
Article on inequalities in health	Understanding and knowledge of issues, relevant theories and views	Slow reading and re-reading, noting own ideas, linking to other reading, questioning the material
Library opening hours	Factual information	Note/memorize for future reference
Technical instructions	Accurate completion of task	Step-by-step reference
Anatomy textbook and diagrams	Informed, factual understanding	Slow and concentrated, re-reading, making notes
Encyclopaedia	Specific definition/information	Specific search under heading
Travel guide	General information	Use of index/contents to locate relevant information

some examples, their possible purpose and the level of reading skill you would require for each.

Consider Table 5.1 for 5–10 minutes. Note in your reflective diary, roughly:

■ *What types of reading you have done this week*

■ *How you went about them, i.e. how did your approach differ in each case?*

From Table 5.1 and the notes in your reflective diary, you can see how you, perhaps unconsciously, employ a range of reading skills. However, you might not be using them as well as you could. For instance, how selective are you in your reading? Do you try and read as much as possible or give close attention to carefully chosen material? When you've finished reading do you understand the content? If not, what do you do about it? Reflect on this in your reflective diary for 5 minutes.

The active reader

Look again at Table 5.1. Most of the reading tasks require some active involvement from the reader. But the two whose purpose is understanding, i.e. the article and the textbook, require several readings, notes/diagrams and an intelligent personal response. Within that, you would consciously have to apply different levels of reading skills:

■ **Skimming/scanning** the material for the gist. You can quickly decide what parts you need to concentrate on, i.e. which sections contain the information you need. Use the layout of the material – contents page, headings, index, tables/charts – to help you.

- **In-depth reading/re-reading** of the denser material. Be prepared to spend time on this and use reference books, e.g. a dictionary for unfamiliar words. Have pen and paper to hand for your notes.

- **Inferring** as you read, i.e. reading between the lines and being aware of the context. You already do this when you read anything: no written material is without context and the same statement in different contexts can have different intent (see Box 5.3). Inference and context are related to subjectivity and interpretation, as discussed earlier.

- **Paraphrasing** important or difficult points and ideas in your notes. In this way you are recording your own understanding of, and response to, the material. Paraphrasing involves you interpreting the material and making sense of it, and this is far more effective than simply highlighting passages of text – not only do you achieve better understanding of, and concentration on, the material, you are also honing your writing skills. The notes you make at this stage may also be the germs of ideas for your essay.

BOX 5.3	*How context can change intent*

Statement: 'I blame the parents'
Context 1: Letter to local paper complaining about vandalism
Context 2: Slogan on T-shirt sold at Gay Pride

In Context 1, we have a straightforward reference to a perceived decline in family values and its effect on society.
    In Context 2, the statement becomes ironic.

Preparation and purpose

Remember: *define and stick to your purpose*. The active reader does this by identifying what they need from their material. Writing these needs down as a series of questions both clarifies and keeps them visible so you don't stray from your purpose. If you are clear about the answers you need, you are less likely to waste time on irrelevant material. However, you will certainly have stray thoughts: note them down for exploration at another time, but stick to the task in hand.

The activity below (10–12 minutes) asks you to read a passage of text, first without and then with identified information needs, i.e. questions. You may then reflect on the effectiveness of your reading in each case.

The passage below is from *Teratologies: A Cultural Study of Cancer* by Jackie Stacey and, as the book's title suggests, begins to place a medical condition in a cultural context. Read it through as you would any text for study.

Heroes

Books about cancer always tell stories. Those who write them offer recognizable narratives of diagnosis, of treatment and of prognosis. Those who read them often do so in search of the comforting hope of survival. Faced with a sudden change in the story of their lives following a cancer diagnosis, many rehearse the possible trajectories which now present themselves through the accounts of those who have been there before them.

There are books written by doctors about 'the facts' you need to know; they tell of the different types of cancer, the typical prognoses and the likely treatments and their side-effects. There are books written by alternative practitioners encouraging a holistic approach to the disease, advising on diet, therapy and a change of lifestyle. There are books written by spiritual evangelists who write of cancer as an opportunity for salvation.

There are also, of course, books written by patients, or their friends and relatives, which offer personal accounts of the experience of living with cancer. If the person with cancer has lived to tell the tale, the story is often of a heroic struggle against diversity. Pitting life against death and drawing on all possible resources, the patient moves from victim to survivor and 'triumphs over the tragedy' that has unexpectedly threatened their life. These are often the stories of transformation in which the negative physical affliction becomes a positive source of self-knowledge. The person who has faced death and yet still lives, who has recognized the inevitability of human mortality, now benefits from a new-found wisdom. Accepting the fragility of life itself, the cancer survivor sees things others are not brave enough to face (or so the story goes). Cancer offers the chance to reassess. It allows the person to pause and to re-evaluate their life: having cancer teaches us that life may be shorter than we thought and that it may be time to decide to live it differently. These are the kinds of wisdoms which are told and retold in books about cancer.

If, on the other hand, the person with cancer dies, the story told is one of loss and of pain, but also tends to be a celebration of their courage and dignity. It may be written by friends, lovers or relatives. Stories of pointlessly shortened lives, lost opportunities, or of medical or industrial malpractice and ineptitude, warn others to try to avoid a similar fate. The late diagnosis, the misread X-ray or the high levels of radiation near nuclear power stations are some of the motivations for authors to tell their stories. But few write (or publish) accounts which tell only of disaster and depression, suffering and unbearable loss. For there is always room for heroism in tragedy and many such stories offer accounts of stoicism and of a fighting spirit. They document the triumphs along the way, even in the event of death.

The market for books about cancer is enormous. Amongst the expanding health and fitness/self-development/New Age and spirituality sections of highstreet [sic] bookstores and the increasing number of publications for sale in health food shops, books about cancer are not hard to find; in fact, they are hard to avoid. Once the news has been broken, books about cancer surface from all directions: they are on every friend's bookshelf, in every shop window. A veritable 'cancer subculture' proves to have been thriving, but, like so many others, it remains invisible until it becomes relevant and then, as if by magic, it seems suddenly all-pervasive. For many people with cancer these books are the starting point of coming to terms with the diagnosis. They are read in the hope of finding a story that fits, of finding a story that offers hope, of even finding a story that ends happily. They are also read for information about the disease or about the treatment: some offer the chance to learn the language of oncology, to understand the principles of chemotherapy or radiotherapy; others educate their readers on the workings of the immune system, the anti-cancer diet or the negative effects of stress on the body. Read all of them and you can become expert in your field, an expert on your particular disease and an expert on yourself.

Given the changes in health cultures in 1990s Britain, the proliferation of this market of 'self-health' cancer books is hardly surprising. As the government cuts in public health provision become the source of endless stories in everyday life (patients returned home prematurely after surgery, beds not available for emergencies, newly equipped wards standing empty because there's no money to staff them, nurses' threats of unprecedented industrial action signalling intense desperation and frustration), people are increasingly encouraged to look elsewhere for reassurance. The introduction of internal markets into the National Health Service in Britain through the National Health Service and Community Care Act (implemented on 1 April 1991) fundamentally changed its principles of organization and management, placing health firmly within a world of competition and consumerism. In these emergent health cultures, where the language of the market has come to dominate ideas about health provision, the scope for appealing to individuals to take charge of their health is ever-widening.

(Stacey 1997, pp. 1–3; reproduced with permission from Routledge.)
Now re-read the passage with the following questions in mind.

1. The author lectures in Women's Studies and Cultural Studies; how is this evident in this passage?
2. Can you think of cancer accounts you have read that fit these descriptions?
3. What links does the passage make in order to suggest that cancer is a cultural and political concern?

The above activity should have helped you to concentrate on the passage in the following ways:

1   The first sentence and the chapter's heading should alert you to the author's approach: it is not conventionally medical; the words 'heroes' and 'stories' imply a cultural rather than scientific discourse. You are startled immediately into a different way of thinking about how society copes with cancer. In addition, it is difficult at this point to tell whether Stacey is using the word 'stories' to

suggest fabrication. She is not, but you will need to ascertain, by the end of your reading, why she uses this term.

2   Thinking beyond the text in front of you, questioning and making connections for yourself are what the active reader must do: here you might pause to list and reflect on accounts of terminal illnesses that you have read. Do they match Stacey's descriptions? (You might also reflect on how illness and disability are reported in the media.)

3   First, Stacey classifies cancer accounts under types of narrative: the 'hero' battles, overcomes/dies/achieves redemption/wisdom, not unlike heroes and heroines in myths, movies and novels. Storytelling, a cultural exercise, helps us to structure the messy, frightening business of cancer, and simultaneously blurs the line between fact and fiction, or if you like, provides us with frames of reference. Second, Stacey links the growing interest in self-health to the NHS's increasingly consumerist and market-led policies of the 1990s. You might need to refer to other documents, e.g. reports, articles and contemporary journalistic commentary, for a richer context here.

Identifying your information needs means you can concentrate on the relevant sections of the passage, and be more precise about your wider information needs. Being selective, i.e. focusing on several well-chosen readings, is essential. However, be prepared for those times when your information needs won't be apparent until you have read the text several times, and occasionally other texts too.

- ■ Your time is limited – you can't read everything
- ■ In-depth reading is time-consuming, but you will understand material better by giving it close attention
- ■ Quality not quantity!

REVIEWING AND RECORDING YOUR READING

Reviewing your reading is a useful way of summarizing what you have learned and ensuring that you have answered your questions as fully as possible. Your review could be recorded with bibliographic details.

Recording the bibliographic details, i.e. the citation, is necessary for your end of essay reference list and to enable you to locate that material in the future. This also applies to audiovisual material – e.g. radio,

TV, videos – and material from the Internet, including how you found it. Brief notes on content and usefulness may be helpful towards future essays. In this way, you will build up an annotated bibliography of material that you have used throughout your course. Such a database can be stored and arranged as you like, but the cheapest, most effective way is on index cards. Box 5.4 shows the possible content of such a record (see also Chapter 4).

BOX 5.4	*Stacey, Jackie (1997) Teratologies: A Cultural Study of Cancer. Routledge, London*

	pp. 1–3, outlines cancer 'genres' and characteristics and relates growth of such books to NHS in enterprise culture/Thatcherism – extensive notes – used for essay on perceptions of terminal illness and treatments; rest of book combines personal experience and sociocultural critique of cancer, treatments and (sexist) attitudes in orthodox and alternative medicine.
	    Related reading – see Cancer Help Centre/Laura K. Potts/Sontag?
	    Uni. library book, class. no?

As an active reader you recognize that:

- reading is work – to be done at a desk, not in an armchair
- you read to learn – keep a dictionary to hand for new terms
- you read at different levels – select material, scan for relevance, read the relevant material in depth
- purpose and preparation help concentration and understanding
- understanding means time spent re-reading and referring to other works
- understanding means engaging with the material, paraphrasing and re-interpreting in your notes
- you must read critically, always being aware of context and that the author has a frame of reference
- you keep records of your reading, recording the bibliographic details and reviewing the contents and value
- your responses and ideas from your reading are the beginning of your essay.

Plagiarism

Keeping records of your reading is essential for your reference list. If you quote or refer to the work or ideas of another person, whether published, broadcast or spoken informally, you must acknowledge your source. To claim, even accidentally, the ideas of others as your own is intellectual theft. If discovered you could fail your course.

Several referencing systems exist. Your university should give you guidelines on which to use in your written work. (See also Chapter 10.)

LECTURES

This section looks at learning effectively from lectures. Many of the principles from reading still apply, but some of the techniques are different.

The role of lectures

You could be forgiven for seeing lectures as the most important part of your course. They are given by the 'experts' and have an air of authority. It follows that you might also see lectures as being wholly the responsibility of the lecturers. Their job is to package and impart knowledge to you, after all.

Neither of these perceptions is true, however. Lectures are certainly important, but their aims are to:

- introduce material (terminology, ideas, theories, a line of argument)
- explain the above
- complement your reading.

Time spent in lectures should be far less than that used for private or group study.

Lectures are of little use unless you participate. As in reading, you must be active. Before the lecture, treat its contents as new terrain. You wouldn't go to a strange city without a map: preparatory reading is like mapping what you are going to hear. During the lecture:

- ask questions
- take notes – effectively.

You will probably recognize the similarity between being an active reader and an active listener. The key is taking responsibility for your own learning. You are being an active student.

Preparation can help understanding and concentration. Think back to a TV documentary you have watched recently. In your reflective diary, reflect on:

- *what, if any knowledge did you have prior to the programme?*
- *either way, how did this affect your understanding and concentration?*

NOTE TAKING IN LECTURES

Lectures can be stressful because you cannot control the pace as you do when reading or watching a video. You end up trying to do several things at once:

- listen
- understand
- take notes.

To get the most out of lectures you should:

- **prepare** – get some idea of the content of the lecture, read background material

- **identify the purpose** in your preparation – note areas on which you want to concentrate and ask questions about

- **summarize** the content of the lecture briefly in your notes – this will help your review

- **review** from your notes and handouts whether you achieved your purpose and plan further reading/discussion.

Unfortunately, this is impossible. You cannot listen and take notes simultaneously. You cannot understand without giving thought to something, and if you're thinking you're not listening. So don't try!

This is why you need to have identified areas for your concentration. You can focus on what is being said and summarize the content in your notes when the lecturer moves on. The act of summarizing means that you interpret and this will help your understanding. It is similar to paraphrasing in your reading notes.

Whatever you do, don't try and write down everything. It is not possible, nor is it the purpose of the lecture.

Styles of note taking

There are as many different ways to take notes as there are students, but they fall broadly into two categories:

- visual
- linear.

FIGURE 5.1	*A visual approach to note taking*

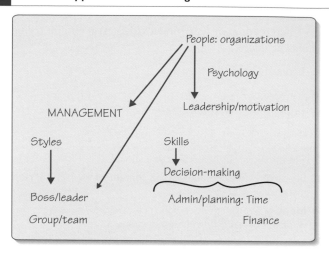

FIGURE 5.2	*A linear approach to note taking*

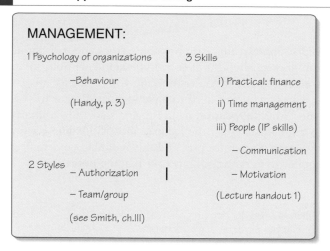

How you take notes depends on you. A visual approach might look like that shown in Figure 5.1.

You are creating a map of your subject, as you did in Chapter 3. This organizes it in your mind and you can note areas for further reading. You can code or highlight areas with different coloured pens so that their importance is obvious.

A linear approach might use headings, indentations and personal shorthand. It might look like that shown in Figure 5.2.

Again, you are arranging the subject, organizing it for your own understanding. This approach can also be highlighted and marked visually. Experiment with styles and adopt the one that suits you, your subject and your needs.

As an active listener you recognize that:

■ you need to prepare for lectures

■ identifying your purpose helps you to focus on the relevant areas during the lecture

■ you will need to ask questions during the lecture

■ you take notes to understand

■ lectures must be supported by reading and discussion

■ reviewing your notes and handouts will help to identify areas for further reading

■ summarizing a lecture is part of the review.

CONCLUSION

Both this chapter and Chapter 3 stress the importance of your role in seeking and using information effectively. Learning takes place not only in the lecture or from reading masses of titles from your reading list, nor is it solely the responsibility of your tutors. Your involvement is the key.

Lecture preparation
Look at your timetable for a lecture that will cover a subject new to you. Note in your reflective journal:

■ the lecture title

■ the subject to be covered.

The day before/of the lecture read briefly round the subject – a chapter or an article. You may not understand it – don't worry. Note in your reflective diary:

■ the reference for the material read

■ the time spent on it

■ your understanding of it, e.g. poor, good.

After the lecture consider in your reflective diary:

■ did your pre-lecture reading familiarize you with terminology, concepts, etc.?

■ was your understanding of the lecture enhanced?

- were you able to make clearer notes?
- were you able to ask questions of the lecturer from a more informed position?
- did you have a better idea of which points you needed to have explained further?

You should have answered positively to some of the above points. It is surprising how a little reading can lay the groundwork of understanding for a lecture on a new subject.

Finally, re-read your pre-lecture material. It should now begin to make sense. It may even round out your lecture notes.

Main points to remember
- Be critical
- Be selective
- Different reading needs require different levels of study and skill
- Prepare for lectures
- Engage with the material.

CHAPTER RESOURCES

REFERENCES

Baron JB, Sternberg RJ 1987 Teaching thinking skills: theory and practice. WH Freeman, New York
Pinker S 1994 The language instinct. Penguin, Harmondsworth
Stacey J 1997 Teratologies: a cultural study of cancer. Routledge, London

Further reading

Cottrell S 1999 The study skills handbook. Macmillan, London

Fairbairn GJ, Winch C 1996 Reading, writing and reasoning: a guide for students, 2nd edn. Society for Research in Higher Education/Open University, Buckingham

Marshall L, Rowland F 1998 A guide to learning independently, 3rd edn. Open University Press, Buckingham

Pauk W 1993 How to study in college, 5th edn. Houghton Mifflin, Boston, MA

6 Group work and presentations

Sian Maslin-Prothero

KEY ISSUES

- Characteristics of groups
- Group work and group dynamics
- Participating in group discussions
- Action in groups
- Tutorials
- Seminars
- Giving presentations

INTRODUCTION

Group work is frequently used as a method of learning in education. This chapter introduces you to some ideas about groups and how they work. The aim of this chapter is to tell you about group work and how to develop your skills for working in groups so that you can get the most out of meetings, seminars and tutorials.

There is increasing emphasis on student participation in learning; the belief is that, through active learning, students are better able to engage in the material being presented and feel more involved in the learning process. There is often an assumption that everyone knows about groups and group work, i.e. what a group is, how a group works, how its performance might be improved and how to personally derive most benefit from a group.

The importance of student participation in other parts of university life is important. You may be asked to become a member of a university body or committee such as a student/staff consultative committee, or represent fellow students at a meeting with the panel from the Quality Assurance Agency to discuss your experience of learning. Becoming a member of any group is an excellent way of developing skills that are key to your development and transferable to other situations.

If you think about it, we all belong to different groups, such as a family, a sports club, a voluntary association or a trade union. Being in a group is how society functions and is therefore a part of all our lives. A group consists of a number of people who meet together to follow a chosen activity. Some groups are more personal and voluntary than others – consider the difference between a basketball team and a seminar group. Groups may form to achieve a specific task, and so group members are expected to work collaboratively.

An effective way of learning is through interacting with other people; it not only gives us the opportunity to hear other people's ideas and thoughts but it also gives us the opportunity to try out and share our own opinions. A group will bring together a wide range of attitudes, knowledge and skills that would not be available if we were working alone. This is one of the advantages of working in a group, particularly when it involves problem solving (such as problem-based learning) or decision making. If all members of a group feel valued and can participate, then there is greater commitment to, and support of, the group and the decisions made. Group discussion can help you develop your critical thinking. However, to be an effective member of any group, you need to understand the process of group work.

CHARACTERISTICS OF GROUPS

Groups have a number of common characteristics:

- a definable membership
- group consciousness
- a shared sense of purpose
- interdependence
- interaction
- ability to cooperate.

Advantages of group work

Reflect on your own experiences of working in a group:
- *What are the advantages of working in a group?*
Jot down your thoughts on a separate sheet of paper.

There are a number of advantages to working in a group, and you might have included some of the following points:

- Sharing the work load:
  - Thinking
  - Problem solving
  - Understanding
- Increased efficiency
- Increased effectiveness

- Mechanism for social support
- Active participation
- Purposeful activity

Disadvantages of group work

There are also disadvantages to working in a group.

- *Can you recall an experience of where a group activity failed?*
- *What do you think was the reason?*
- *What do you think might be some of the disadvantages of working in a group?*

  Jot down your thoughts.

A group might be unsuccessful for a number of reasons, some of which are listed below:

- Poor group dynamics
- Lack of communication
- Task set is not completed
- Not all members of the group participate
- Group members feel isolated
- Group members compare themselves with others
- Gossiping between group members
- Dominance by an outspoken member.

Therefore you need to understand why groups need to exist, and develop strategies for ensuring they are successful and work. As highlighted in the advantages of groups, a group can bring together a range of skills and knowledge that an individual on their own would not have. This can be used to the advantage of the group in achieving tasks. For the group to be successful, all the group members need to feel that they are a part of the group and that the group values their contribution.

GROUP DYNAMICS

In order for a group to be both effective and efficient, you need to have a mix of personalities. There are a number of different roles assigned to members within groups – these roles are usually unconscious. The role you play in a group will depend on your personality and on the reason for the group existing. Belbin (1981) identified eight key roles for an effective group. These are:

- Company worker – practical person who organizes the group and makes any tasks manageable
- Chair – co-ordinates the group and ensures that all contributions are heard
- Shaper – pushes the group and encourages the group to complete the task
- Plant – the creative source; provides the group with ideas
- Resource investigator – liaises with people outside the group and explores new ideas
- Monitor evaluator – the critic who finds the faults in arguments
- Team worker – the individual who holds the group together and supports group members
- Completer finisher – the perfectionist who ensures that the group meets any deadlines.

One person can take on more than one role in a group. It is important that there is balance between each of the roles in the group if the group is to remain effective.

Having looked at the different roles in a group, which would be your preferred role?

Becoming a team player

Our previous experience of working in a team can affect how we approach to working in a new group. In order to be effective the group may need to go through a number of stages before it becomes a functioning team. Teams can go through four stages:

1   **Forming (orientation).** This is usually a positive stage when you are anticipating working with a new group of people. You might be slightly anxious at the thought of meeting people and wondering whether you will be able to successfully complete the task set.

2   **Storming (dissatisfaction/conflict).** At this stage you might experience some uncertainty regarding the effectiveness of the group – if the team does not seem to meet your or others' expectations. There may be disagreements as some members appear to be engaging with the group and activity more easily than you.

3 **Norming (resolution/cooperation).** This is where the team begins to settle down and functions more effectively, because you have addressed any conflict and negotiated how to cooperate.

4 **Performing (productivity).** This is where the team is working well together, where members feel that they are able to express themselves and that the task can be achieved through combined effort.

In order for the team to develop and move forward you need to move through these stages. This can be facilitated by agreeing ground rules during the forming stage.

Ground rules

Participating in group discussions enables us not only to learn from others, but also to develop our own thoughts and beliefs about a subject. If the group is to be successful it is important that the group members meet and agree ground rules. Ground rules are a set of guidelines that the group acknowledges and adheres to each time it meets. Having ground rules allows each member of the group to know what is expected of them.

Imagine you are meeting in a group for the first time. Jot down the sort of ground rules that would be important to you. Keep these and refer to them when you are asked to identify ground rules.

You might have identified some of the following as important:

- Confidentiality
- Being tactful, considerate and respecting others' opinions
- Punctuality
- Being supportive:
  - Sharing knowledge
  - Not 'putting down' others
- Not being distracting:
  - Keeping noise levels down
  - Not interrupting
  - Sticking to the point.

The use of ground rules allows each member of the group to know what is expected of them, as well as of other members of the group. There may also need to be agreed sanctions for members who break any of the ground rules.

MANAGING A GROUP

The last section examined the development of the group and roles of individuals in a group. Prior to looking at how you can contribute to a group discussion, you need to understand about managing a group. A successful group will be purposeful, without the need for teacher intervention. The two main factors in managing a group are:

- group tasks
- group maintenance.

Group tasks

The task or tasks of the group relate(s) to its purpose, structure and activities. These need to be clearly defined – e.g. group composition, members' roles and tasks, group management, ground rules (these are discussed in more detail above), study requirements (seminar presentations, assignments, assessments), deadlines and preparation for meetings.

Group maintenance

This is all about creating a climate that encourages discussion and debate. It can be achieved through the group members being accepting of and cooperative towards each other, particularly when there are conflicts of opinion or personality clashes. Active participation makes group sessions enjoyable, as well as producing an excellent opportunity for learning.

The amount of time spent on the maintenance of a group will vary; it is particularly important in the early stages of a group's formation.

Group meetings

In order for the group to be effective, everyone needs to be committed to it. This means attending group meetings. By not turning up for a pre-arranged meeting, you are not sharing the commitment to the group and are letting your colleagues down.

The group needs to have a focus, i.e. a 'frame of reference' – the subject the group is going to discuss or a task the group has to achieve. For example, your lecturer has asked you to find out about the principles of asepsis as part of a problem-based activity. In order to develop your understanding of asepsis you have to expand your knowledge, through thinking, brainstorming ideas, reading or discussion. Through sharing the topic with others you will be able to keep sight of the frame of reference, and move forward by utilizing the opinions of others, as well as by cultivating your own.

Groups go through stages of development before performing successfully. If a group meets on a regular basis then it can build on the information gained at previous meetings, thus enabling the conversation to become more advanced and sophisticated. The group will also change and develop over time, from its initial formation, through conflict, cooperation and finally task completion.

Group discussion

Many students gain support from a group. Not only are you developing your own academic skills, you are contributing to others' learning as well. It can be a comfort to find that some students have similar thoughts to you, while others may offer a different way of examining an issue. For example, imagine you have been asked to read a complex article in preparation for a group seminar. You read the article but you can only make sense of the abstract – the rest of the article makes no sense to you. When you meet for the seminar, you discover that some of your colleagues were equally baffled. However, some of the group understood parts of the article. Through group discussion and cooperation you will be able to grasp and make sense of the article.

The group can provide support in other ways, such as sharing articles or learning skills. We all experience difficulties in our lives and, through sharing these difficulties, we can help each other and make the ordeal of learning less stressful.

What do you do if you don't want to participate in the discussion, possibly because you are too shy or because you are afraid that your colleagues might think what you have to say is daft? Remember that discussion is there for everyone's development, not only those who appear to have no fear of expressing their thoughts and feelings. In this situation, don't be afraid to make an observation – what appears quite simple to you might be just what another colleague needs in order to make sense of the subject. Another important point to remember is that we all feel anxious about expressing ourselves; even experienced people feel inadequate and anxious about contributions they make to debates.

As discussed at the beginning of the section on group dynamics, we all have different roles in a group and, so long as you participate by actively listening, you are contributing to the group discussion.

WHEN THINGS GO WRONG

There will be times when things go wrong in a group. The most important thing is to maintain a climate of cooperation. This can be

achieved by involving the whole group in identifying the problem
and then in resolving it.

Hostile members

This problem can occur in both small and large groups. Examples
include overt hostility, aggression, point scoring and inappropriate
humour, all of which can hinder the success of the group. It is important to acknowledge any hostility when it occurs. If you feel you need
additional support, call on other group members to support you
when you tackle hostile members.

Avoiding difficult situations

This is when members of the group avoid a specific issue by being
disruptive, withdrawing from group activities or trying to change the
subject. You need to recognize when this is occurring and vocalize
your thoughts – remember, communication is essential if the group
is to be successful. You may find that the group relies on the same
person to make all the difficult decisions. If this is the case, do ensure
that you support this member where appropriate.

Dominating members

There will be occasions where some of the group dominate the conversation and prevent others from participating. If someone, such as
a lecturer, is facilitating the group, you might see it as their responsibility to control the group. However, each member of any group has
a role and responsibility for regulating the group – more so if specific
ground rules were agreed; so don't be afraid to manage unruly
members. Your backing will be appreciated, not only from your
colleagues, but also by the facilitator.

SELF-HELP GROUPS

You can establish an informal self-help group to achieve specific
tasks, such as revision for examinations or writing an essay (see
Chapters 2 and 7). Don't wait for someone else to do this – set up the
group yourself.

- Listen to other group members
- Appreciate others' contributions
- Communicate
- Don't let the group down

- Give the group time to achieve its aims
- Enjoy yourself.

ACTION IN GROUPS

There are other methods of learning used to help develop your understanding of a subject. Experiential learning means learning by doing, i.e. you learn from experience. This refers to learning through everyday experiences in life and work – being aware of them, then thinking and reflecting on your experiences (see Chapters 11 and 13).

Interactive teaching and learning methods include:

- one-to-one discussion
- buzz groups
- brainstorming
- role play.

These interactive teaching methods involve active participation by group members. The thought of participating in these different methods of learning can be quite daunting but in reality they can be an excellent way of learning and developing other skills. Not only do you learn about the subject being covered, you also learn about members of your group.

One-to-one discussions are frequently used as ice breakers. A group is divided into pairs and each pair is given a task. The task might be to find out about each other and then to introduce your partner to the rest of the group. Or pairs are asked a specific question, which they then have to discuss and feed back to the whole group. This type of activity also helps you to develop your listening skills.

Buzz groups are often used when there are large groups. The group is divided into subgroups of four or five students. Each subgroup is given a specific topic to discuss, which they feed back to the whole group. This is a useful way of involving the whole group and of encouraging quieter members to contribute to a large group, through small group discussion.

Brainstorming is a way of generating creative and different ideas. The group is given a problem, and a few minutes to think of possible solutions. The group is then invited to contribute these ideas, and all ideas are welcomed and recorded. The aim is to generate as many ideas as possible. Once these have been recorded, then the group can use the points for discussion. Role play is a teaching and learning technique used for developing skills such as interpersonal communication or empathy, or for dealing with difficult issues. The facilitator will set the scene and explain the exercise. Students will be invited to participate by acting out specific roles. The participants will have their role explained; there may even be a script. Those students observing the role play will be asked to contribute by observing what is going on in the role play and, when invited, commenting on the interactions that occurred. Don't be embarrassed, and do have a go at participating in role play. It is important that everyone is deroled on completion of the exercise. You can reflect and comment on your experience of what you felt and understood.

These different methods of teaching and learning can be linked back to Chapter 2, where you identified your preferred method of learning. Your preferred learning style might not be to participate actively because you find this rather threatening. But do consider that the very act of participating can allow you to learn – experiential approaches can be far more interesting and stimulating than more formal methods of teaching and learning.

TUTORIALS

Tutorials may occur on a one-to-one basis or with a small group of students meeting with their tutor or lecturer. The overall aim of a tutorial is to learn from a small-group discussion and to develop your ability to listen, evaluate, criticize and argue. Therefore you need to be prepared for your tutorial; if you have been asked to prepare for the tutorial, i.e. to read an article or bring an outline for an assignment, then do so.

Tutorials can end up becoming mini-lectures from your lecturers; you might not learn much if this occurs so don't be afraid to contribute and even challenge your lecturer. As Chapter 5 highlighted, lecturers don't know everything; by contributing you will develop your argument and other critiquing skills.

SEMINARS

Occasionally you will be asked to present a seminar; this is a popular teaching and learning strategy in nurse education. This section will examine points you need to consider prior to undertaking a seminar. A seminar involves giving a short presentation on a chosen topic, usually drawing on a variety of sources, for approximately 10–15 minutes. Students may be asked to present on their own or in a small group and the presentation is followed by a general group discussion.

Initially, this can seem overwhelming for many students; however, preparation is the key. First of all, ascertain from the facilitator exactly what they want you to cover. Don't be tempted to do too much; do only what you were asked to do and you will be surprised how quickly the time goes. The function of your presentation is to stimulate debate among the group. You might find it helpful to have an overhead projector acetate, a Microsoft PowerPoint slide or a photocopied handout prepared for your audience, with the main points of your seminar written down. Remember that the subject will be familiar to you because you have prepared the seminar, but not to your colleagues. Keep your presentation simple and be prepared to explain or illustrate certain components for your colleagues. Following the initial presentation, it is part of your responsibility to engage your fellow students so that a general discussion ensues.

Preparing a seminar

■ What?
  – What are you expected to present?
■ How?
  – How long have you got for your seminar?
  – Is it an individual or group presentation?
  – How is it going to be assessed (formative or summative assessment)?
■ Who?
  – Who are you presenting to?
  – Who will undertake the assessment (teacher, peer or both)?
■ Finally, do you need to submit an outline of the seminar to your lecturer?

If you are presenting as a member of a group seminar, there are further points that need to be considered, if it is to go well, relating to group dynamics. You need to ensure that the work is shared equally between group members and that everyone knows what they are supposed to be doing during the seminar presentation.

If there are key points to be made in the seminar, write them down on a whiteboard or flip chart. These can be used to focus the discussion following the seminar. As presenter, you also need to control the group and make sure that people do not deviate too much from the topic under discussion. Finally, summarize the main points raised at the end of the seminar.

Seminars allow you to participate in your teaching and learning. They will help you to learn how to find, collate and present information, and then receive feedback from your colleagues. The skills you develop from seminar presentations are transferable and can be used when preparing other assignments, such as essays.

PRESENTATIONS

Presentations are a way of sharing information with colleagues. They can be used as a way of sharing factual information with a particular audience and are employed as a form of assessment on many courses.

The following are characteristics of a good presentation:

- The information is clear and relevant to your audience
- Progress is logical
- There is visual as well as aural presentation
- The audience is responsive.

For a presentation to be successful you must prepare in advance. The following will provide you with the necessary information to prepare a presentation.

Preparing a presentation

- Why?
    - Why are you presenting?
- Who?
    - Who is your audience?
    - What is the size of the audience?
- What?
    - What is your aim?
    - What do they already know about the subject?
    - At what level shall you pitch it?
    - What shall you include?
- How?
    - What learning method should you use?
    - What are the key points?
    - Are you there to inform, persuade or amuse?
    - How long have you got?
- Where?
    - Where will you be doing the presentation?
    - Do you have any choice?

- Understand what you are to present (know your subject)
- Structure the presentation
- Prepare notes to guide you
- Identify visual aids to support your demonstration

Structure

Preparing for a presentation is similar to writing an essay: you need to know your subject through researching it (see Chapter 3 on using the library and Chapters 8 and 9 on writing). Once you have the information, you need to structure your presentation. As with preparing an essay, you need an introduction, main theme and conclusion. The introduction introduces the audience to what you are going to be discussing, the main body expands and develops the topic, and the conclusion is when you pull the whole thing together and summarize the key points.

You should have a main theme or idea that you follow – having aims and objectives (see Chapter 1 for definitions) can help guide you and your audience through the presentation. The development of the presentation should be logical; your message should be clear and to the point. If you are going to change direction in your presentation, tell your audience that you are moving on to another area so that they can understand where you are going.

Finally, you should conclude by summarizing the main points, telling the audience what you have already told them, and linking it to your aims and objectives.

Delivery

Once again, preparation is the key. You should be well rehearsed and know what you are going to be talking about. The use of motivators can attract individuals to your presentation, encouraging them to attend. These can come in the form of a question or a picture, and it will help the audience to identify the relevance of your topic to their personal experience.

Remember, you are going to be communicating with the audience using the spoken word, supported by non-verbal clues such as your facial expression or the clothes you are wearing. You need to decide from the start whether you are going to present formally, with little or no interaction with the audience. In this situation, ask the audience to leave questions for when you have completed your presentation. Alternatively, you may choose an interactive session where the audience participates with activities, group work or discussion.

With thorough preparation, and brief notes to guide you, you can interact with your audience by maintaining eye contact and using appropriate gestures. Use the clues they provide to guide your presentation. For example, if they look puzzled, perhaps the definition of an unusual term, or a more detailed explanation, is required.

As anyone involved in public speaking will verify, giving a presentation can be a nerve-racking experience. Ensuring that the room is ready, with the correct seating arrangements, lighting and equipment, will help make you feel much better. Finally, be enthusiastic – enthusiasm is contagious, and you will find that your audience will be eager to listen and engage.

Equipment

You can use audiovisual aids to support and enhance your presentation, for example:

■ Overhead projectors (OHP)

■ Slide projectors

■ Television and video recorders

■ Tape recorders

■ Whiteboards

■ Flip charts

■ Microsoft PowerPoint

■ Computer.

Know what equipment is available, know how you are going to use it, and make sure that it works. Tables or graphs (see Chapter 4 on information technology) can act as a focus for the group participants. However, it is important not to provide too much information for your audience because this will not give them the opportunity to understand what is being said, reflect and ask appropriate questions. Use an audiovisual aid only if it can enhance your presentation, not just for the sake of it.

Audiovisual aids

■ Do be prepared

■ Do have the right equipment (and make sure that it works)

■ Do know how to operate the equipment

■ Do use keywords

■ Do use large, bold writing/print

■ Don't use more than a few audiovisual aids

■ Don't have too much information

■ Don't obscure the view

■ Don't write/print in small writing

■ Don't panic. If something goes wrong, take a deep breath, find your place, and continue with your presentation

Questions

As mentioned above, let your audience know at the beginning of the presentation when you are prepared to answer questions. Try to anticipate the most likely questions based on your presentation, and prepare for them.

When asked a question, be sure you have understood what you are being asked. If it is unclear, ask for the question to be repeated or rephrased. If you are unable to answer the question, be honest and say so. You can invite other people in the audience to answer, if they have knowledge of the subject. When replying, make sure your answer is clear, relevant and to the point.

CONCLUSION

This chapter has looked at group work and the different types of group you might encounter when learning. It has looked at how groups are formed, how groups work, the role of different group members, how to organize group meetings, how to participate in a group and what to do if things go wrong. The last part of the chapter looked at presentations and how to prepare and present to colleagues.

Bear in mind the following:

- There is an increasing emphasis on group and team working
- Group work involves active participation
- To be successful, individuals have to adopt different roles in a team. You will probably have preferred roles
- To be successful a group must communicate and act on decisions made
- Be prepared for a group to change and develop over time.

Before moving on, take some time and record in your learning diary:

- your preferred role in a group (based on Belbin's eight key roles) and why you prefer this method of working
- whether you have experienced conflict of opinion in a group and, if so, how this was resolved.

CHAPTER RESOURCES

REFERENCES

Adair J 1986 Effective team building. Gower, Aldershot
Belbin RM 1981 Management teams – why they succeed or fail. Butterworth-Heinemann, London

7 Examinations and revision

Heather Wharrad

INTRODUCTION

Examinations seem to create more anxiety for students than any other form of course assessment. In this chapter you will learn strategies for preparing and revising for examinations and for optimizing your performance in the examination itself. Examinations are brief snap-shots of what you have learned from a period of study; by planning for them at the start of the course (and during it) you can minimize the stress you feel on the day of the examination. This can't guarantee good results but it will give you the best chance of success.

PREPARING FOR EXAMINATIONS

You will almost certainly have taken examinations before.

Think back to the last examination you took. How early in the course did you start to prepare for it? Did you feel confident on the day of the examination that you were fully prepared?

The chances are that you did not give much thought to the examination when you started your course – it probably seemed a long way off. When it came to the day of the examination you were probably wishing that you had been better prepared.

BE ACTIVE NOT PASSIVE

Anxiety about an impending situation can lead people to be passive and 'just let it happen'. You should avoid leaving all your preparation to near the examination date. The more actively you plan and prepare for the examination at the beginning of (and throughout) the course, the more likely you are to succeed. Rhetorical comments such as 'Well, it's not in our hands' and 'What's in the exam's just a lottery' contribute to the feelings of helplessness experienced by students who feel that the lecturer is controlling the situation. Indeed, this principle applies equally to preparation for any type of assessment or placement – the more active and engaged you have been in preparing for the event, the more successful and rewarding it will be. One of the first tasks should be to check on the format of the examination paper(s) and the type of questions you will be given.

TYPES OF EXAMINATIONS AND QUESTIONS

Unseen examinations

Traditional unseen examinations (the student does not 'see' the question paper beforehand) are still the most common form of examination used, although the types of question on the papers can vary considerably. Some of the commonly used types of question are described in Box 7.1.

BOX 7.1

Multiple-choice questions
These consist of a 'stem' – this is the question – and usually four or five branches – these are the answer choices. The student has to select one answer that, relative to the other choices, is correct.

Example
The normal number of pairs of human chromosomes in cells is:
a. 48 b. 47 c. 46 d. 23

Fill in the gap questions
These questions require the student to enter the most appropriate word or phrase that fits into a gap in a statement. Sometimes students are given a list of responses to choose from.

Example
Fill the gap in the sentence below with the correct name of the procedure described.
[tracheonomy; tracheostomy; tracheotomy; bronchiostomy]
A _____ is an artificial opening into the trachea at the level of the second or third cartilaginous ring, which is kept patent by the insertion of a metal or plastic tube.

Short-answer questions
Students write short answers to a number of questions, the answers being anything up to one page in length. This type of question requires students to make

concise, succinct points and they may be asked to draw a diagram to illustrate the answer. You should be clear about how many marks are allocated for these questions and obtain guidance from your lecturer about the length of answer expected, and whether bullet points, flow diagrams or illustrations are acceptable. Preferably, you should be given some 'model answers' as a guide.

Examples
 (i) Describe three criteria that promote wound healing
 (ii) Outline five factors that might cause an inaccurate measurement of oral body temperature.

Long-answer or essay questions
Essay questions require students to write at length about the questions posed. Marks are likely to be awarded on the structure of the essay – does it have an introduction and conclusion, does it flow logically – as well as on the content and inclusion of major points (see Chapter 9).

Open-book and seen examinations

Open-book (where you can use books during the examination) or seen examinations (where you see the questions before the examination and can therefore prepare your answers prior to the examination itself) are not as easy as they sound. In an open-book examination you will be penalized for copying down information word for word from the books; indeed, there are issues of plagiarism to consider too (see Chapter 5). You will need to be very familiar with the texts that you are expected to use so that you can go straight to relevant sections, otherwise you will spend a lot of time in the examination searching for the information.

In both these types of examination, you will be given marks for how you analyse the information and use it to develop a logical argument, and not for merely describing the information.

An open-book examination allows you to rely on the printed word for details; what it is testing is not your memory but how you can use the information to make a rational argument or analyse an issue.

A seen examination gives you time to gather relevant material and evidence and to think about the presentation and structure of your answer. Accordingly, the examination markers will expect you to present a more considered answer than in an unseen examination.

Practical examinations

Many nursing courses now incorporate examinations of practical nursing skills into their assessments. The objective structured clinical examinations or OSCEs are one type of practical assessment of nursing practice competence (Harden 1988, Nicol and Bavin 1999).

During an OSCE students rotate around a number of time-limited stations. These may comprise a patient scenario or situation devised to assess particular skills, for example taking blood pressure, assessing respiratory function or carrying out cardiopulmonary resuscitation, or the student might be required to complete a short written assessment or interpret some clinical results. An examiner is present at each station, observing and scoring the performance according to predetermined objective criteria. The scoring systems used for OSCEs vary; an example scoring sheet indicating the criteria for a urine-testing station is shown in Figure 7.1.

On-line examinations

Web-based course tools such as WebCT (www.webct.com) and Blackboard (www.blackboard.com) and software such as Questionmark (www.questionmark.com) enable examinations to be put on line. The advantage of computerized examinations is that marking is done automatically within the computer application and a list of marks can be generated very quickly. Questions tend to be multiple-choice or fill-in-the-gap formats.

Viva voce examinations

Viva voce examinations are normally used to supplement other forms of assessment, such as dissertations. They normally take the form of interviews, where students are questioned about selected sections of a piece of written work. Usually a viva is used to convince examiners that a student is the 'owner' of a piece of work on the basis that the student can talk about it with familiarity and a certain amount of conviction. Vivas have often been used to help make decisions about borderline cases in degree award classifications and, less frequently, as a form of course assessment.

EXAMINATION PREPARATION

At the start of the course

All students are supplied with course information, including learning outcomes or objectives, at the start of the course. You should also obtain information about the course assessments. Make sure you get as much information about the format of the examination (such as the number of papers, the length of the examinations and the types of question in the examination paper) as you can. This will help you to plan your revision and practise appropriate types of question when the time comes. It is also worth checking on the Internet for

| FIGURE 7.1 | *Example scoring sheet for an OSCE urine testing station* |

Outline

The student will demonstrate the correct procedure for testing urine using labstix, identify any abnormal finding and give a possible cause and rationale for the abnormal finding.

Introduction

Greet the student and give the following information:

Assume two patients have provided a urine sample. The samples X and Y are here. Demonstrate how you would test the urine, identify any abnormal findings and state a possible cause with a brief rationale for the stated cause.

Time

8 minutes (1 min intro, 5 min practical, 2 min feedback).

Equipment

Urine sample, labstix, recording sheet.

Action	Score
Student identifies urine to be tested and prepares the record sheet	
Checks time	
Dips stick fully but briefly into the urine samples	
Taps excess urine back into the container	
Reads stick against reagent colours on the chart on bottle at approximately correct times	
Writes down findings on record	
Appropriately disposes of urine and used labstix and washes hands	
Identifies any abnormal finding(s)	
States a possible major cause of such abnormality	
Gives rationale for the stated cause	
TOTAL	

Key: Performs adequately = 1, Attempted but inadequate = 0.5, Not performed = 0

Signature: Student _____

Examiner _____

web pages relating to the subject you are studying. More and more online nursing databases and sources of evidence for practice are being developed. NMAP is a computer gateway to Internet resources related to nursing (www.nmap.ac.uk) and provides only high-quality resources that have been through an academic review process. Adding useful, high-quality web addresses to your list of favourites on your computer at this stage may save you time later when you are supplementing your notes, revising or looking for practice examination questions (see Chapter 5).

During the course

You will save time during your revision period if you follow the points listed below. Many students fall into the trap of thinking that they understood a teaching session until it comes to revising the material and then the concepts seem less clear. They then use their valuable revision time trying to make sense of the material, and they may have to seek assistance, perhaps from a lecturer – again, this can be very time-consuming. By reviewing the lecture notes soon after the session you will ensure that you know whether you need to spend a little more time understanding the material and adding to your notes. A good test of your comprehension of the material is to try to write down a few key points to summarize the material covered in the session. You can then spend 5–10 minutes reading through these key points during the rest of the course. If you have had other course work marked, use the lecturer's feedback to identify gaps in your knowledge or in what ways you need to improve your writing style.

- Make good notes and make sure they are complete (see Chapter 5)
- Review and summarize lecture notes as soon after the lecture as you can (see Chapter 5)
- Spend time understanding the material
- Read through summaries and key points regularly
- Learn from feedback from other assignments
- Underline and make marginal notes in your textbook or on handouts
- Link theory and practice components (see Chapter 14)

You will save yourself time during your revision period if you have underlined and made marginal notes in your textbooks or on handouts when you review and summarize your notes. This way, if there are points you need to check through again you will be able to go straight to the relevant sections of the textbook or handout. Even at this point you could give some thought to when you will begin your revision period. Some courses build a revision period into the timetable but you need to consider whether this is an appropriate length of time for you. At least provisionally planning your revision time at this stage means you are less likely to put off the revision planning as the course comes to an end, and you become more anxious about the impending examinations.

The final point in this section concerns relating the theory and practice components of the course. Information is often much easier to remember when its use and relevance is seen in a 'real situation'. If you have a period of nursing practice, look at your course notes to see where there are links with what you have practised and what you have seen in practice. Add marginal notes to remind yourself of these links (see Chapter 14).

At whatever stage you are at in your course, use the checklist below to find out how prepared you are for an impending examination.

Have you:

- Read through the module objectives?
- Checked the length and format of the examination?
- Got your notes up to date and complete?
- Supplemented notes using texts and websites?
- Made marginal notes about links with practice?
- Obtained practice examination papers?

REVISION TECHNIQUES

Your revision time is precious. It is a time for consolidating and organizing in your mind the material you have studied. You should not allow yourself to start looking at new information. Retaining a positive attitude at this stage is very important. Do not allow negative thoughts to enter your head; this will affect your concentration and reduce your efficiency.

There is no universal revision technique that suits everyone. The method you choose will depend on your personal preferences in the way you work and the type of course you are revising. You should also consider the format of the examination paper before you plan your revision strategy. A multiple-choice paper will cover a greater breadth of material than will a paper offering a choice of essay questions. This may influence whether you revise the whole course or focus on a number of key topics.

Planning your revision timetable

When planning your revision timetable, work out exactly how much time you have available – be realistic. You won't be able to work solidly for every hour of your waking day. Work out how long you will need for sleep, meals and recreation (see Chapter 1). It is important to allow yourself regular breaks in your revision time. Many students find it useful to draw a timetable grid like the one shown in Figure 7.2. Break down your study material into manageable chunks (the smaller the better, but this will obviously depend on the time you have available to revise) and place them into the time slots in the grid.

Adapt the grid shown to suit your own study style. For example, if you can only maintain your concentration for 40–60 minutes, have 1-hour time slots rather than the 2 hours shown. You may prefer to vary the topics from session to session within a day to retain your interest and concentration, or you may prefer to complete a whole topic before moving on to the next. If you find that your timetable slips, don't abandon it completely (and don't feel a failure either). Modify the timetable in whatever way is necessary to get you back on track.

Strategies for remembering information

The best strategy for remembering information is not to rely totally on short-term memory. Instead of soaking up the material like a sponge and regurgitating it during the examination, it is better to think it through and analyse it, make judgements about it and think how it relates to nursing skills or practice settings. By performing these analytical and reflective processes, you are more likely to commit the information to your long-term memory, which is much more reliable than your short-term memory. There are, however, strategies you can use for remembering stages in a process, sequences of event or lists of items.

Association and visualization

If you have been making lists of key points or bullet points and have been reviewing them during the course you will probably find that you can visualize the information on the page or card on which they are written. Processes or events can be drawn as flow charts, timelines or diagrams to explain a sequence of events or to link information. Mind maps are a useful way of remembering the relationships between concepts and ideas (Buzan and Buzan, 2000). Some examples of mind maps can be found at the Open University learners-guide website (http://www3.open.ac.uk/learners-guide/learning-skills/revision/min_map.asp) and the mind map shown in Figure 7.3 is taken from an article by Hendry and Farley (2003). Visualization approaches

FIGURE 7.2   *A revision timetable*

Week 1

	Monday	Tuesday	Wednesday	Thursday	Friday	Saturday
8.30–10.30	Anatomy	Microbiology	Revision group tutorial	Developmental psychology	Swimming	
11.00–13.00	Anatomy	Microbiology	Social policy	Developmental psychology	Health psychology	Health psychology
14.00–15.30	Play squash	Practise MCQs	Social policy	Developmental psychology	Health psychology	Shopping
16.00–17.30	Microbiology	Practise MCQs	Practise questions	Developmental psychology	Health psychology	Practise questions
19.00–20.30	Microbiology	Meet friends	Tennis	Practise questions	Club	Practise questions
21.00–23.00	Pub			Concert		Pub

Week 2

	Monday	Tuesday	Wednesday	Thursday	Friday	Saturday
8.30–10.30	Nursing theory	Nursing theory	Revision tutorial (lecturer)	Read revision notes	Exams	
11.00–13.00	Nursing theory	Nursing theory	Practise questions	Read revision notes	Exams	Relax
14.00–15.30	Play squash	Practise questions	Read revision notes	Practise questions	Exams	
16.00–17.30	Nursing theory	Practise questions	Read revision notes	Practise questions	Exams	
19.00–20.30	Nursing theory	Swimming	Tennis	Practise questions	Relax	
21.00–23.00	Pub			Meet friends		

FIGURE 7.3   *Example of a Mind Map (adapted from Hendry and Farley 2003)*

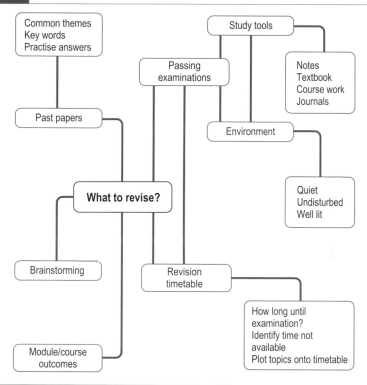

such as these can be a very powerful memory aid: we use them all the time in everyday situations such as visualizing what is in your wardrobe when choosing a new item of clothing or visualizing a room when choosing wallpaper or a new piece of furniture. Some examples of these ideas are given in Box 7.2.

Other ways of remembering your notes are to link topics with everyday objects or group things together verbally. Some people make up a story that incorporates the information they are trying to remember.

Using mnemonics, for example, the well-known mnemonic Richard Of York Gave Battle In Vain, ensures that nobody forgets the colours of the rainbow, and the order in which the colours appear (Red, Orange, Yellow, Green, Blue, Indigo, Violet).

Certain types of information can be remembered in the form of acronyms, for example NATO (North Atlantic Treaty Organization) or OMNI (Organising Medical Networked Information) and rhymes (e.g. to remember the number of days in the months many people recite '30 days hath September, April, June and November . . .').

BOX 7.2	**Example 1**

Example 1
Sequence of movement of blood through the systemic circulation:
Capillaries → Venules → Veins → Right atrium → Right ventricle → Lungs → Left atrium → Left ventricle → Aorta → Arteries → Arterioles → Capillaries

Example 2
Key stages in the birth of the National Health Service (NHS) 1900–1950:
1909 – first call for an NHS attributed to Beatrice Webb
↓
1942 – Beveridge report – health care one of three basic requisites for a viable social security system
↓
1944 – White paper (*An NHS*) – equal access to medical and allied services
↓
1946 – NHS Bill of March 1946 proposed nationalization of voluntary and municipal hospitals
  – NHS Act became law on 6 November steered by Minister of Health Aneurin Bevan
↓
1948 – birth of NHS on 5 July

Can you think of a mnemonic to help you to remember the names of the different white blood cells in the body? These are neutrophils, basophils, eosinophils, lymphocytes and monocytes.
  How about:
Basil Eats Live Newts Mondays

During your course you will be spending time in practice, or you may be learning practical skills in a skills laboratory. Students often find it easier to remember information if it is linked to practical skills or to other practical experiences. When you are in practice or learning these practical skills think about the theory you have been doing in the classroom. The association you make between the theory and practice may help you to remember more of the information in an examination.

Repetition

Memory depends on repetition. Whether it is learning a technique or remembering certain facts, the more times you practise a technique or read through information the more likely you are to remember it. Try the following ways:

- Write out a number of times
- Repeat out loud
- Record on to tape and replay
- Read, recite then check.

Only the last of these needs some explanation – 'read, recite then check'. The best way of carrying out this exercise is to cover each set of key points in turn, then expose only the headings relating to your key points. Recite all the key points you can remember relating to that heading, uncover the key points to check how many you have remembered. If you are satisfied with your answers, move on to the next heading. If you missed out some important points, repeat the process until you get it right.

Try these repetition methods now with notes from a recent teaching session. Rather than relying on just one of the methods listed above, alternate between them, this will help to retain your interest.

Self- and peer-testing

It is crucial to test yourself on what you have learned and revised; only then will you know how much you have understood and remembered.

- Write out half a dozen headings then jot down the key points under each subheading
- Make up some practice questions yourself or, better still, ask for some past papers or example questions from your lecturers
- Many textbooks now have self-test or self-assessment questions at the end of chapters – check your own textbooks

Self-testing requires self-discipline. Be strict with yourself – the more you test, the more you remember. Many students find great benefit in working with friends or groups, discussing topics and testing each other (see Chapter 6). This can create a very supportive environment in which to work.

Four key words underpin a successful revision strategy – remember the first letters, PQRS, to remind you what they are:

- Planning
- Question practice
- Repetition
- Self- and peer-testing.

The P represents planning early and throughout the course. Q refers to question practice as often as you can. R is for repetition – the more times you practise a skill or go through the course material, the more likely you are to remember it. S is for self- and peer-testing. This will give you confidence in the course work you do understand and will highlight any gaps in your understanding.

The night before and on the day of the examination

The night before the examination, check your timetable and organize pens, pencils and any other instruments you may need for the examination. Reading through your key points will not do any harm but cramming at this stage is probably not helpful. Check your timetable again when you wake up and give yourself plenty of time to eat a meal and travel to the examination. Try to fill the time before the examination with practical things rather than dwelling on what questions might come up on the paper. Arrive at the examination in good time, take some deep breaths and don't decide that everyone else looks far more confident than you do.

DURING THE EXAMINATION

General advice for all types of examination

Read right through the paper (for up to 5 minutes) and jot down any facts that occur to you as you read. This will help you to relax and give you confidence. Read through the instructions for candidates carefully and underline important instructions, such as the number of questions you have to answer in each section or that you have to write your answer on separate sheets.

Underline the key instructions on the front sheet of the exam paper below:

University of Trentham

School of Nursing and Midwifery

Semester 4 Examination

Time allowed: 2 hours

Candidates should attempt to answer all questions in each of four sections. Answers should be written in the answer book provided.

Write each answer on a new page.

You should have underlined '2 hours', 'all questions', 'four sections', 'answer book' and 'new page' as the key instructions.

Spend a little time identifying what precisely each question is asking. Some of the 'action' words that might be used are shown in Box 7.3, with brief definitions of what they mean. Underline these and other key words in the question.

BOX 7.3

Analyse – explain the relationships between . . . (sometimes more vaguely stated as 'Comment on')

Assess – determine the importance or value of . . . (sometimes more vaguely stated as 'Comment on')

Compare – explain the commonalities (similarities) and differences between . . . (more emphasis on commonalities)

Contrast – explain the commonalities and differences between . . . (more emphasis on differences)

Critique/Critically analyse – explain relationships and provide evidence for and against the relationships

Define – state precisely and succinctly the meaning of . . .

Describe – write what something is like, how something happens or what the main characteristics are

Discuss – write a logical argument on . . . (may require you to analyse, critique, evaluate, explain . . .)

Evaluate – for something that has already happened . . . use evidence to estimate its importance

Explain – give reasons for . . . or say how something works

Illustrate – use examples to demonstrate a point, e.g. statistics, diagrams, graphs

Justify – say, giving valid evidence, why something is true

List – provide a column or row of relevant items, with no description

Outline – point out the main features of . . .

Prove – use logical steps and evidence to establish the truth of . . .

Review – look back over something and comment on its value

State – write down the main points

Summarize – write down the main points without all the detail

Trace – follow the pathway of . . .

Underline the key action words in the exam question shown below:

Section 4 (25 marks)

Answer all the questions

1. Explain what is meant by immobility (2 marks).

2. Discuss the effects of immobility on three body systems (10 marks).

3. Describe, with rationale, measures that may be taken to prevent/alleviate the effects you identify (10 marks).

4. List three devices that might help a client who is immobile to carry out activities of daily living (3 marks).

You should have identified the key 'action' words as underlined below. Also, note carefully the number of marks allocated to each question, this determines how much time you should spend on each part.

Section 4 (25 marks)
Answer *all* the questions

1 <u>Explain</u> what is meant by immobility (<u>2 marks</u>).
2 <u>Discuss</u> the effects of immobility on <u>three body systems</u> (<u>10 marks</u>).
3 <u>Describe, with rationale</u>, measures that may be taken to <u>prevent/alleviate</u> the effects you identify (<u>10 marks</u>).
4 <u>List three</u> devices that might <u>help</u> a client who is immobile to carry out activities of daily living (<u>3 marks</u>).

Re-read the questions and answer your best question first. As you work through the paper, jot down any thoughts that come into your mind about answers to other questions. If you don't write ideas down immediately the chances are you will forget them. If you miss out part of a question, meaning to return to it later, mark it clearly, so it stands out and you don't forget to answer it. Leave some space at the end of your answer in case you want to add another point later. Check your answers, and check that you have answered all the questions. If at the last minute you find you have forgotten to do a whole question, or you have run out of time, write an answer in note form with subheadings (similar to your revision key notes). You may scrape a few extra marks this way.

Essay questions

Spend at least 5 minutes planning your answer before you start to write your essay. Jot down main ideas and important ideas as bullet points in rough. Write a brief introduction to your essay. In the introduction, refer to the question being asked. This will serve two purposes. First, it signposts the essay for the examiner and, second (and just as importantly), it will ensure that you focus on all parts of the question being asked. Many students make the error of writing a good examination answer on a similar but wrong topic and get no marks at all. After reading the question and recalling some of the key information in your mind, ask yourself 'Am I recalling the correct information for this question?' Don't allow yourself to waffle or over-answer – you won't get more marks and you might run out of time.

You are likely to get more marks for two half-answered questions than for one answered and one unanswered. While you are writing your answers, think about the following points:

- Are you dealing with the major issues?
- Are you writing simply and directly to the point?
- Are you writing legibly, without misspellings and grammatical errors?
- Are you making drawings bold and clear?

Your plan should help you to write down the points you want to make in a logical order. You should always end your essay with a conclusion, drawing together all the points you have made in the main body of the answer.

Multiple-choice examinations

Multiple-choice examinations require as much revision preparation as any other type of examination. There is a tendency for some students to do less preparation and to rely on guesswork, rather than putting in the revision and practice time to allow them to make rational and logical judgements about the answers. You should remember that multiple-choice questions allow coverage of a greater breadth of material than other types of questions and require detailed knowledge and logical thought as well.

Multiple-choice examination papers are often marked mechanically and inappropriate pen marks could result in incorrect marking. Read the instructions carefully. Make sure that you don't mark two answers. If you mean to go back and decide on which you think is the correct response at the end of the examination – don't forget. Indicate these questions clearly to remind yourself.

Scoring systems in multiple-choice examinations vary. You should be clear about these before the examination and, ideally, you should have practised your technique. For example, if there is what is called 'negative marking' for incorrect answers, then you cannot make a guess at an answer you are unsure of. On the other hand, if there is no such penalty, it is reasonable to make a guess at the answer.

It is particularly important to read every multiple-choice question very carefully. Sometimes there may be a qualifying phrase that completely changes the meaning of the questions. You should also watch out for 'double negatives'. To clarify the meaning, try to translate double-negative statements into positive ones, for example 'not true' would become 'false', and 'not lacking' becomes 'having'. You can see in the examples in the box below how easy it is to be confused by a double negative and give a totally wrong answer.

Underline negative words, such as 'not', and qualifying phrases, in the questions below:

Which of the following is not an uncommon systemic symptom of inflammation?
a. paralysis
b. shock
c. nausea
d. fever

Uncontrolled diabetes mellitus is associated with which one of the following:
a. a decreased urine output
b. low blood glucose levels
c. high blood glucose levels
d. high levels of insulin in the bloodstream

Which of the following is false. Respiratory rate:
a. in a newborn baby is faster than in an adult
b. cannot be altered consciously
c. is controlled by the medulla
d. increases during exercise.

You should have identified the words underlined below as those that are key to the meaning of the question. Misreading these words will totally change the meaning of the question and lead to you giving a wrong answer.

Which of the following is <u>not</u> an <u>uncommon</u> systemic symptom of inflammation?
a. paralysis
b. shock
c. nausea
d. fever

<u>Uncontrolled</u> diabetes mellitus <u>is associated</u> with which <u>one</u> of the following:
a. a <u>decreased</u> urine output
b. <u>low</u> blood glucose levels
c. <u>high</u> blood glucose levels
d. <u>high</u> levels of insulin in the bloodstream

Which of the following is <u>false</u>. Respiratory rate:
a. in a newborn baby is <u>faster</u> than in an adult
b. <u>cannot</u> be altered consciously
c. <u>is</u> controlled by the medulla
d. <u>increases</u> during exercise

Online computer delivery is becoming more commonplace for multiple-choice examinations. Computer packages, known as virtual learning environments, such as WebCT and Blackboard allow tutors to set up tests and examinations relatively easily and they do have the advantage that marking is done by the computer quickly and automatically. Preparation for these computerized examinations should be the same as for a paper-based examination. However, you should make sure you have used the computer package before the day of your examination so that you know how to log into it, have read the instructions about how to navigate around the package and understand the instructions about how to submit your answers.

COPING WITH EXAMINATION ANXIETY

It is perfectly natural to feel nervous and anxious about examinations. It is the nature of this type of assessment that creates this stress. Examinations are a one-off assessment requiring our best performance on the day. When you have worked hard throughout a course, you want to do yourself justice by performing well and achieving a high mark.

One of the physiological responses to stress is to produce more of the hormone adrenaline (epinephrine). Adrenaline puts us into the 'fight or flight' mode – we can either face the challenge and give it our best shot, or we run away from it. Whatever the challenge, be it public speaking, running a race, performing a solo or taking an examination, the extra 'nervous energy' can be used to enhance performance. By remaining focused and positive about the examination you will find that your heightened state of anxiety will enable you to concentrate for longer periods of time and remain more focused on your work. During your period of revision there will be a great temptation to use this energy for 'displacement' activities, such as tidying 'that' cupboard because you just can't put up with it any longer (even though it's been just as untidy for the last 6 months). You must try to avoid such displacement activity and focus on your revision. The other activity to avoid is panic conversation with your peers. This can waste a lot of time and will only serve to exaggerate negative thoughts. Remember, you have a revision timetable to stick to. If you feel you are getting over-anxious then talk to a lecturer or a student counsellor about it. They will be very experienced in dealing with these problems.

- Some anxiety is natural and will enhance your concentration and performance
- Channel your nervous energy into focusing on the task in hand
- Eliminate negative thoughts, remain positive and active
- Don't disrupt your normal eating, sleeping and recreational routine too much: this can worsen symptoms of stress

AFTER THE EXAMINATION

Before the sense of relief you feel after the examination, you will naturally go over the paper in your mind and discuss your answers with your peers. Try not to dwell too long on these 'post-mortems', especially if you have other examinations to do. It is important to keep your morale high. You have probably done better than you think.

Ten tips for passing examinations:
- Do some work regularly throughout the course
- Be active and positive, not passive and negative
- Start working towards the examination NOW
- Manage your stress levels
- Test yourself regularly
- Ask for help sooner rather than later
- Plan a timetable for study and revision
- Don't stop all your recreational activities in the run up to the examination
- Get an overview of the course material as well as the detail
- Make links between theory and practice.

CONCLUSION

This chapter has given you a range of strategies to help you to prepare for examinations. By building some of these strategies into your study plans, you will increase your chances of being successful and reduce the stress and work-load in the days before the examination.

CHAPTER RESOURCES

Web resource links

The following links also provide some useful tips on coping with examinations and how to develop good revision techniques:

Effective revision 1999. Liverpool Hope University, UK: http://www.livhope.ac.uk/gnu/stuhelp/revis3.htm

Revision and exam technique. University of Bradford, UK: http://www.brad.ac.uk/acad/civeng/skills/revexam.htm

Revision and examinations Open University, UK: http://www3.open.ac.uk/learners-guide/learning-skills/revision/pages/index.asp

REFERENCES

Buzan T, Buzan B 2000 The mind map book, revised edn. BBC Consumer Publishing, London

Harden RM 1988 What is an OSCE? Medical Teacher 10(1): 19–22

Hendry C, Farley A 2003 Examinations: a practical guide for students. Nursing Standard 17(29): 48–53

Nicol M, Bavin C 1999 Clinical skills learning: teaching and assessment strategies. In: Nicol M, Glen S (eds) Clinical skills in nursing: return of the practical room? Macmillan, Basingstoke

Further reading

You may find the following texts and articles helpful in developing your revision strategies and improving your examination technique:

Acres D 1994 How to pass exams without anxiety: every candidate's guide to success, 3rd edn. Northcote House, Plymouth

Gibbs G 1994 Improving student learning: through assessment and evaluation. Oxford Brookes University, Oxford

Hendry C, Farley A 2003 Examinations: a practical guide for students. Nursing Standard 17(29): 48–53

2 DEVELOPING YOUR WRITING SKILLS

8 Information seeking for assignments

Abigail Masterson

KEY ISSUES

- ■ Literature searching skills
- ■ The World Wide Web
- ■ Purposeful reading

- ■ Evaluating sources and the written word
- ■ Primary and secondary sources

INTRODUCTION

As nurses and midwives we must continually update ourselves on what is being done and discovered so that our practice is underpinned by the best knowledge available. In order to write meaningfully about a topic you need to be able to extract the right sources and review the available literature – text and World Wide Web based – in a systematic, organized and purposeful way.

Such skills do not come naturally but need to be learned and practised. Reviewing the literature is not just something you do as a student – being able to evaluate what you read in journals, books and on the Internet is fundamental to knowledge-based practice. Having read and worked through the activities you should be able to take appropriate notes and make decisions about the relevance and usefulness of different sources.

The principles apply to reviewing literature for all types of assignments whether they are conventional essay style, case studies, reports or dissertations.

PREPARATION

Preparation is the key to success in everything and it is important to start researching for assignments early. If you leave your preparation to the last minute, you may find that your colleagues have all got there first and that few of the key texts are left in the library. If you are going to make best use of the resources on the web, this too takes time. Many web sites now offer full-text journal articles and research reports but often these require you to be registered with the appropriate company and/or to pay to download them. Prices in 2004 were as much as £20 for a full-text article from the Journal of Advanced Nursing, although your university library and/or your professional association library may offer some full-text journals on-line for free. Planning your time carefully and making the best use of your local library facilities is much cheaper!

- Find out the opening times of the libraries that you will need to use. Remember that during holiday times libraries may be closed or have reduced opening hours. Many libraries allow free or cheap access to the World Wide Web but often such sessions have to be booked in advance.

- Ask your librarian if your institution subscribes to a full-text online journals service such as Athens, and if so how you can register to use it: are there any forms you need to fill in? Will you require a password? Will your password allow you access from your PC at home or do you have to use a library PC?

- Identify how long you will allow yourself for getting together resources, how long for reading and how long for writing and editing. It is often tempting to get completely caught up in reading and gathering together more and more references. Be sure to leave yourself time to actually read all the information you have collected properly and to write the assignment.

MAKING THE BEST USE OF YOUR RESOURCES

It is always worth taking some time to identify the most appropriate and relevant resources (see Chapter 3 for more details). Such resources should also include people who may have an interest in the area, or with whom it would be useful to talk through your ideas. For example, if you are working on an essay about the nursing care of a patient with diabetes it might be useful to talk through your ideas with a patient who has this problem, a representative of an interest group such as the British Diabetic Association and/or the local diabetic nurse specialist. If you are writing on a professional issue such as account-ability and midwifery practice then you might find it helpful to make an appointment with the senior midwife in your clinical area, or your mentor, to get their perspective, and to contact the Nursing and Midwifery Council (your regulatory body) and/or your professional association/trade union. If there are several of you all working on a similar topic or area it may be helpful to work together. You can then share resources and try out your ideas on each other. Also you will not have to spend so much time individually in the library searching the literature, surfing the web and photocopying articles.

PLANNING

It is important to spend time thinking about your assignment before you start your literature search and talk to your patient/client if it is a case study. This thinking should involve clarifying the topic, jotting down your thoughts and listing all the questions and issues that occur to you. This type of thinking should ensure that your reading becomes purposeful rather than haphazard. It is crucial to focus on exactly what is required. It is often tempting to read things just because they are interesting rather than being absolutely clear that they are relevant. Equally, if you are not sure of your focus you may waste time going off on tangents and getting together loads of material that is not really relevant. (See Chapter 5 for further tips and hints.)

 Imagine you have been asked to produce a review of the nursing literature in relation to health and the implications for health promotion in children's nursing practice. Note down the key issues you would want to include.

Your list might look something like this:

- What is health?
- Models of health
- Attitudes to and perceptions of health in children and their families
- The influence of culture on health and health beliefs
- Developmental needs in relation to health
- Health education and health promotion strategies for children and their families.

This list would give a useful framework to help you select what sort of resources you need to use, what key words you need to use for your literature search and some of the points you might want to make in your discussion. You may find it helpful at this point to refer back to Chapter 3 in which getting the most from your library is discussed in more detail.

RESEARCHING SKILLS

Researching, or collecting material and resources together for your assignment involves being systematic and organized. It is vital to record carefully accurate details of what you are reading, however time-consuming or irritating this may seem initially. When carrying out literature searches it is particularly important to note down the full reference, including the year of publication and the name and place of the publisher. In edited books it is necessary to record the names of the editors and the names of the authors, page numbers and titles of the individual chapters you wish to refer to. Some journals unfortunately do not include the details such as year of publication and volume and issue numbers on every page. Unless you write these on the copy of the article at the time, even though you have a photocopy of the article you may waste valuable time re-finding these details later.

Recording references

Some people use index cards to record this sort of information because they are small enough to be carried around easily but large enough to contain the essential information that you need. In addition, they can be sorted into alphabetical order, which saves time when you come to write up your references and bibliography. Each book, chapter, article or report that you read should be recorded on a separate card. Increasingly, people are using personal computers to store this type of information and there are now several software packages available to help you do this, e.g. Reference Manager, EndNote or Database. These allow you to type in details as you go, much as you would on a card index, to insert references into the text of your assignment and to create a list of your references either as a separate document or added to the end of your assignment. Most will also allow you to save references you have found on the Web. This can be complicated; however if you think you are going to take your studies further or are working on a very big project such as a dissertation, taking time to learn how to do this could be worthwhile (see Chapter 4 for a further discussion).

For example, the information that should be recorded for a book is:

Bellman L 2003 Nurse-led change and development in clinical practice. Whurr, London

For a journal article:
Albers L 2003 Reducing genital tract trauma at birth: launching a clinical trial in midwifery. Journal of Midwifery and Women's Health Mar/Apr 48(2) pp. 105–110

For a chapter in an edited book:
Masterson A, Mitchell L 2003 Developing competences for advanced nursing practice. In: McGee P, Castledine G (eds) Advanced nursing practice, 2nd edn. Blackwell Publishing, Oxford, pp. 31–46

And for an Internet resource:
Author(s); date of publication; Title of article. Title of Serial/Monograph [type of medium] volume number (issue number): pagination. Availability statement. [Date of accession, if needed].

International Federation of Library Associations and Institutions 2003 Library and Information Science: citation guides for electronic documents. Available on line at: www.ifla.org/I/training/citation/citing.htm pp. 1–3 [accessed 28 November 2003]

Some parts of the generic format are not always applicable to all electronic publications, of course.

With text-based resources, it is often useful to note down where the reference is kept. For example, did it come from a particular library or did you borrow it from someone? Noting down the class number and accession number can also help speed things up if you need to find the same reference again. If you are using web-based resources be sure to note down the full web address so that you can locate the reference again should you need to. The subject matter of the reference should be noted too, along with the key points of argument or information it contains.

For example if you were writing an essay about disability, a useful reference which you might come across in your literature search would be Barnes C, Mercer G 2003 Disability. Polity Press, Cambridge.

Your card on Barnes and Mercer (2003) might look something like this:

BOX 8.1

Describes the historical developments in the disability literature internationally and from a wide range of disciplinary perspectives such as sociology, social policy and politics. Argues strongly for a social model of disability and points out the impact of the pioneering studies carried out by disabled activists and the growing politicization of disabled people around the world in challenging the established belief system and thus service provision. The nature of the social oppression, exclusion and marginalization experienced by disabled people is explored in relation to family life, reproduction, education, employment, leisure, cultural imagery and politics. Disability is also considered in relation to gender, race, social class and age. Through these analyses a wide-ranging critique is offered of traditional 'professional' understandings of and approaches to disability which they suggest instil dependence and prevent disabled people from living more autonomous lives.

It is helpful to note down any direct quotes that you may want to use in your writing. For example Barnes and Mercer (2003, p. 12) offer this useful explanation of the social model of disability:

> In the individual model, 'disability' is attributed to individual pathology, whereas the social model interprets it as the outcome of social barriers and power relations, rather than an inescapable biological destiny. . . . Moreover instead of an individualistic regime of rehabilitation and personal care services, the 'disabling barriers' diagnosis suggests wide ranging social

changes coupled with alternative forms of service support and provision.

A review of research into managing urinary incontinence in older people might lead you to the 2003 article of Mandy Fader and colleagues, 'Management of night-time urinary incontinence in residential settings for older people: an investigation into the effects of different pad changing regimes on skin health' in the *Journal of Clinical Nursing*, vol. 12(3), May 2003, pp. 374–386 and your card might look like this:

BOX 8.2

- The aim of this study was to examine the effects of different pad changing regimes on skin health.

- Improvements in technology have resulted in highly absorbent products, which may be worn all night, but the effects of prolonged pad wearing on aged skin are unknown.

- A crossover research design was used.

- Patients were randomly allocated to one of two pad changing regimes: a frequent pad changing regime (every 4 hours) or a less frequent pad changing regime (every 8 hours). Each regime lasted 4 weeks and was followed by the alternative regime.

- Skin measurements were taken twice during each regime.

- Measurements indicated that skin was 'wetter' in the less frequent pad changing regime.

- Five patients developed grade 2 pressure ulcers during the less frequent pad changing regime, but none in the frequent pad changing regime.

Includes lots of other useful references to follow up.

The key is being succinct but informative. You may find it helpful to keep the question and your initial brainstormed plan close to you while you are reading to make sure that you extract only relevant information and do not get completely snowed under with notes.

THE WORLD WIDE WEB

The Internet is a network of networks that connects millions of computers from all around the world using the telephone system. Once you connect to it (log on) you have access to millions of sources of information. You can use the Internet to access general and specialist information, send messages to people around the world and participate in discussion groups. No one owns or controls the Internet and the infrastructure can be somewhat shambolic.

The World Wide Web consists of millions of magazine-style pages containing text and images, plus multimedia elements such as sound samples, animations and video clips. Many institutions and individuals now have websites. Commercial companies use them to tell you about their products and services and to allow you to place orders. Educational institutions provide information about their courses and often a range of interactive self-directed learning materials such as lecture notes, tutorials, online quizzes and video clips of clinical procedures. You can access online bibliographic databases such as CINAHL, MEDLINE, the Midwives Information and Resource Service (MIDIRS), the British Nursing Index (BNI) and Athens. (Some of these require you or your institution to be registered and can only be accessed using a password.) There are news services provided by organizations such as the BBC and CNN, online newspapers such as the *Guardian* and *The Times*. Even professional magazines such as the *Nursing Standard* and *Nursing Times* have an online version. Charities, support groups and pressure groups use websites to give details of how you can help them, what support is available for patients and families and information about the cause of the condition with which they are involved. Individuals with particular interests use websites to share their knowledge – this can range from obscure hobbies and interests to advances in cancer care (see also Chapters 3 and 4).

There is a great deal of information devoted to health, nursing, midwifery and related topics. Much of this is currently American but the amount of information from the UK and other countries is growing rapidly. 'Surfing' the web is a lot like using a multimedia CD ROM but the material you are looking at could come from anywhere on the Internet. Pages are connected together by hypertext links, enabling you to move about by clicking on underlined text or highlighted images. For example a page on human immunodeficiency virus (HIV) and acquired immune deficiency syndrome (AIDS) might have links to pages on drug treatments, complementary therapies and support services. You can also go directly to a particular page if you know its address.

Internet search tools

Searching the Internet can be frustrating at first but with a little practice it is possible to locate information quickly and efficiently. There are three types of Internet search tool that can help: search engines, web directories and subject gateways.

Search engines gather websites automatically – there is no human intervention and no quality control. You will get lots of results but many may not be relevant to your needs. You have to create your own search terms and so it is always useful to look at the help pages provided as each search engine works in a slightly different way and knowing how best to organize your search terms can save time and greatly improve your search results.

Web directories use human editors to some degree but quality control is still variable.

Subject gateways provide access to evaluated websites so the quality is generally higher.

Try out the following Internet search tools:

Google – http://www.google.com

Yahoo – http://www.yahoo.com

Subject gateway to nursing, midwifery and the allied health professions – http://nmap.ac.uk

Each offers different features. Follow their instructions on how to refine your search. For generic search engines such as Google, UK-specific search facilities are best avoided. They usually promote UK-based domain names ending 'uk' e.g. xxx.co.uk over American-based '.com' sites regardless of content and may therefore exclude UK sites hosted on US computers.

Discussion groups

Most Internet service providers (ISPs) provide the means to subscribe to discussion groups – special interest groups where you can follow or contribute to a discussion, ask questions and network. Useful UK nursing and midwifery related discussion groups are sci.med.nursing; sci.med.midwifery and alt.support.student-nurse.

SELECTING SOURCES AND DECIDING RELEVANCE

It is much easier to read something if you have some idea about what it is going to be about and are sure that it is likely to be relevant or useful. Research reports are usually prefaced with an abstract. This is a summary of why the study was done, what it is about and what the main findings and conclusions were, and also includes key words. In book chapters this sort of information is usually included in the first paragraph or introduction. In this book, for example, the introduction states quite clearly what the contents of the book are, what order they are covered in and who is likely to find it helpful. In journal articles this information may be included in the introduction and/or the abstract if there is one.

BOX 8.3

If you were carrying out research into the postnatal support required by parents, the following abstract might well catch your eye:

Simons J, Reynolds J, Mannion J, Morison L 2003 How the health visitor can help when problems between parents add to postnatal stress. Journal of Advanced Nursing 44(4): 400–411

Background. Caring for a baby can provoke or intensify discord between parents, with adverse effects on their own well-being and their parenting.

Aim. The aim of this study was to appraise evidence obtained from 450 mothers on the quality of the parents' relationship during the postnatal period and the value of support provided by health visitors in cases of discord.

Design. The health visitors were based at nine clinics in an outer London borough, and had been trained on a 4-day course (the Brief Encounters course) to screen mothers for relationship problems at the 6–8-week check and to offer support (supportive listening, practical advice, referral) if problems were revealed. Data on relationship quality were obtained by a self-report screening scale completed at the 6–8-week check and again at the 12-week visit for immunizations, when the scale was included in a self-report questionnaire on help received from the health visitor. Intervention records kept by the health visitor showed what form any support had taken. Some 6 weeks later, 25 of the 82 mothers offered support, and their health visitors, were interviewed about their experience of the intervention.

Results. One in five mothers were identified as having a relationship problem at the 6–8-week check. Most were offered support. One in five of the 351 mothers who completed a questionnaire at the 12-week visit reported receiving support in improving their relationship. The follow-up interviews showed that most mothers valued this support. Responses to a questionnaire completed by health visitors showed that most were enthusiastic about its benefits.

Conclusions. A 4-day training course for health visitors enabled them to screen for relationship problems during the postnatal period and to provide support when required in a way that was valued by mothers. Most health visitors were enthusiastic about the value of the intervention in improving their contribution to family welfare.

Well-constructed books will also have a list of contents and an index. It is useful to scan both of these to see whether or not there is any explicit reference made to the topic you are studying. Then turn to the relevant pages and scan them quickly focusing particularly on headings and subheadings in order to see whether or not there is anything useful there.

PURPOSEFUL READING

Once you have done this to check relevance and appropriateness it is important to read the whole thing right through, carefully and thoroughly. This section builds on the reading skills that you worked on in Chapter 5. All the time you are reading it is important to keep stopping and reviewing what you have read. The purpose of reading is to weave new ideas and information into your own thinking in order to reach a new level of understanding about a subject or topic. It is often useful to mentally ask yourself questions as you read. Some examples are given in Box 8.4.

BOX 8.4

'Is this an account of a research study or someone's views and opinions?'

There are many interesting, well informed journal articles, web-based materials and books written by well known authors but if your assignment asks you to review recent research then it would not be appropriate to include them. If, however, you are reviewing the literature in order to ascertain the current understanding of a phenomenon such as spiritual aspects of care, then such opinion articles, if well justified and referenced, would become relevant.

'How recent is the work/ideas being discussed?'

There is often a gap between writing and publishing of as much as 2–3 years. Journal articles tend to reach publication more quickly than books, although the work they report on may be a few years old. Articles can be published on the Web instantly. Some areas of nursing and midwifery are changing very quickly so the information in books may be almost out of date as soon as it is published. Or the recommendations may have been superseded by more up-to-date knowledge. That alone does not necessarily mean that it should be discarded. It depends on the question or topic area that you are trying to address. For some topics a historical context may be very important.

For example, if you were analysing a nursing model such as Dorothea Orem's or Sister Callista Roy's, it would be important to give depth and richness to your analysis to note how the model had changed over time and the modifications and refinements that have been made in response to the critique of other theorists and practitioners. Similarly, if you were writing an historical account of changes in the education and preparation of nurses and midwives, or developments in nursing and midwifery interventions, then some quotes from original textbooks and journal articles would provide a rich source of examples.

'What country does the author come from and what country are they writing about?'

Increasingly, libraries stock books and journals from many other English speaking countries and many British journals contain articles from authors working in other countries. Some things will be common to all countries, others will not. Drug names, for example, are sometimes different between the USA and the UK, the length of education and the way nurses and midwives are taught is different in Australia, the law is different in Scotland and England. Consequently it depends on what you are writing about whether such contributions are relevant. If you are writing about developments in the field of mental health nursing it may well be relevant to draw some cross-national comparisons. If however you are discussing the merits of different wound dressings you need to be sure you are comparing like with like; and a discussion of legal issues regarding the rights of people with a learning disability would need to be confined to a particular country.

'Why is the author/researcher writing what they are writing?'

If a midwife researcher has been sponsored by a baby milk company to conduct research into patterns of breast feeding then they may have been encouraged to show bottle feeding in a positive light. Similarly, a patient/client education leaflet about the treatment of leg ulcers that has been sponsored by a wound dressing manufacturer will probably present the manufacturer's own products as particularly helpful.

'What are the points the writer/researcher is making? Are these points validated and justified by other literature or research?'

In some areas of nursing and midwifery practice there are differences of opinion about the 'right' way to intervene or support patients/clients with particular problems or the right way to organize things. For example, in areas such as pressure area care and wound healing there is a lot of apparently contrary evidence; and there is a growing body of research and opinion articles supporting midwifery-led care where the same midwife sees the woman for all her care both antenatally, during labour and following birth, yet there are other reputable studies that advocate team midwifery.

'Do I agree with the inferences and conclusions the writer has made?'

In research studies in particular it is extremely important to read carefully all the titles or captions that accompany tables, charts and diagrams. Well constructed work should flow logically and the foundations for the conclusions that are eventually drawn should be apparent throughout.

'Do I understand it?'

The unclear or overwhelming will usually make sense if you take the time to read what it says. It is helpful to be able to change your reading speed so that you can read the easy bits fast and skim over them but take your time during the difficult bits. It also depends why you are reading. If there is a key resource it may be vital to spend a lot of time reading one article or book chapter to pick up every single point and nuance that it contains. Alternatively if you are attempting to get a broad perspective on the range of opinion in a particular area then skim-reading several sources may be more beneficial.

Unfortunately, some of the academic writing in nursing and midwifery is very jargon ridden, is written in American English and is unnecessarily complicated, which can be very confusing, off-putting and frustrating at first. Specialists always develop their own language because it gives them extra power in analysing their subject in a detailed and systematic way. As you study subjects in greater depth and become a 'specialist' yourself, you will gradually find yourself using the same technical language without even noticing. For example you may already find that you are beginning to talk about 'therapeutic relationships' and 'obs', 'MIs' instead of heart attacks and to feel comfortable using words such as 'symbolic interactionism' and 'dysphasia'. Using technical language is not meant to annoy or be exclusionary and elitist but to develop new ideas; new words are part of the process of developing knowledge about a subject.

'How does this work fit with the rest of what I have read?'
It is important to be clear about the chronological order of developments. There is no point in rejecting someone's work because it doesn't allow for some development that occurred 10 years after it was written. Ideas are refined and developed over time. For example, good practice in care of the elderly settings in the 1970s in the UK involved a focus on maintaining safety and fostered dependence on nursing staff whereas nowadays good care is seen as that which upholds the right of older people to be independent and to take risks. Similarly, some diversity of opinion is beneficial and informed debate is healthy and necessary but it is important to be clear about what the differing stances are and the merits or otherwise of a maverick opinion or finding.

'How does this work fit in with my own experience?'
It is often useful to think about occasions and events in which you have come across similar patients/clients or problems to those you are reading about and to consider how the author's point of view or description fits with your own.

'What are its strengths and limitations?'
Being able to evaluate the merit of a piece of work and the arguments or information that it contains is crucial. It is often useful to evaluate what you are reading in relation to your own practice and nursing as a whole.

NOTE TAKING OR PHOTOCOPYING

You might be wondering whether it is most useful to take notes, or just to print off web pages and photocopy every text source you need. All are probably vital. Printing off web pages can be very time-consuming and therefore expensive. If possible, download and save the information on to a disk to read later. (NB. some sites – particularly commercial ones – prevent you from doing this.) Photocopying is quick and is particularly useful for journal articles but can get very expensive. With books there are restrictions about how much you are legally allowed to photocopy. Consequently it is useful to learn how to take appropriate notes.

If you are using photocopied articles then you may find it useful to highlight key words, points and phrases. If however you are likely to use the same article again for something else then it may be better just to underline the salient bits in pencil which can then be rubbed off when you are finished. If the book or article is your property you may find it helpful to jot down in the margins comments, thoughts, questions and examples that came into your mind as you read it.

Note taking forces you to think as you read because you have to decide what to write down and clarify your interpretation of what you are reading. It also forces you to stop day-dreaming as you read. Notes should not merely be a summary of what is in the text. The secret of note taking is to identify key words, points and phrases with regard to your purpose. The notes you require for a complex, key text will be very different from the notes you write to summarize an article that you just happened to read in passing. Different people acquire and store information in different ways but generally you need to think 'What is this about?' and 'What do I need to remember?'

Effective note taking depends on identifying and arranging key points to suit your own thought pattern and way of working. Some people find that drawing spider diagrams and flow charts is helpful; others develop their own shorthand. (See Chapter 5 for further information on note taking.) The important thing is that your notes should make sense to you when you come back to read them several weeks or months later. Also, you may not be able to borrow that particular book again or get back to that library so you need to make your approach as effective as possible so that one reading is enough. Conversely, there is little point creating pages and pages of notes that just describe and reiterate what you have read. You do not need to take notes on everything that you read, as some reading should just be about broadening your knowledge base and familiarizing yourself with different ideas and different points of view.

You will need to develop some kind of filing system for your notes so that you can find what you want when you need it. It is also useful to record and remember which databases and libraries you have used, what you have already read, and any conversations with tutors/facilitators. It is important to keep your notes safe – don't carry them all around with you or you might lose them and have to start all over again.

THE INFALLIBLE 'GOD' OF PRINT

There is a tendency to be seduced into believing that if something is in print it must be true and the author's interpretation must be right. However, it is healthy to develop a bit of scepticism about everything that you read and to develop skills in evaluating the importance of a piece of work to your purpose, i.e. writing an academic essay or research-based report. This is particularly important in relation to web-based material. Journal articles and books usually have to go through some form of review process prior to publication and there are therefore some safeguards about the quality of the material. Anyone who is prepared to pay a small fee for web space can publish on the Internet.

Books and articles are written for different purposes and different audiences. Textbooks are intended to provide general introductions to specific areas of interest such as the care of particular patient/client groups or subjects such as sociology and physiology. The intention of such books is to provide a straightforward, broad understanding. Specialist books aim to provide more depth and detailed analysis of defined areas. There are also growing number of books produced only in an online format – see, for example, *The Internet and IT for Busy Nurses and Therapists*, available free on line from the European Institute of Health and Medical Sciences at the University of Surrey – or that are produced in an online and hard copy format – see, for example, Masterson A, Humphris D (eds) 2000 *Developing New Clinical Roles: A guide for health professionals*. Churchill Livingstone, Edinburgh.

The *Nursing Times* is the mainstream of popular nursing literature in the UK. It is written in an accessible style, has a huge circulation and is published weekly. The *Nursing Standard* aims to help nurses keep up to date with clinical developments and is also a popular weekly publication. Both the *Nursing Times* and *Nursing Standard* have panels of expert referees who review the articles submitted for publication to ensure that a particular standard is achieved but the intention is not to produce academic, scholarly work. *Professional Nurse* is a monthly journal, which also aims to provide articles that are informative but readable and practice-orientated for clinical nurses. The *Nursing Times, Nursing Standard* and *Professional Nurse* are available for sale in most major newsagents.

Midwives is a monthly journal that is sent free to all members of the Royal College of Midwifery (RCM). It is the official journal of the RCM and contains regular features on topics of interest to midwives, some research papers and review/opinion papers. It is accompanied by a monthly news and recruitment supplement and, twice yearly, a peer-reviewed scholarly supplement called *Evidence Based Midwifery*. The *British Journal of Midwifery* is a monthly peer-reviewed journal that is very readable and has a very large circulation. It publishes topical papers from student midwives, midwives and other professionals, including doctors and legal experts. *Practising Midwife* is also a popular British journal, published monthly, which aims to address current clinical issues. For example, a recent issue included articles on Birth Centres and postnatal contraceptive advice.

The Association of Radical Midwives publishes a quarterly journal, *Midwifery Matters* for its members, which offers a vehicle for its lay and midwifery members to discuss issues related to the values of the Association, which campaigns against the un-necessary medicalization of childbirth.

Two of the major international journals that are useful for UK midwives are *Midwifery* and *Birth*. Both are available on subscription, highly respected and peer-reviewed. *Midwifery* aims to enhance quality of care for childbearing women and their families. It publishes research papers from all over the world on issues as wide-ranging as domestic violence in Australia and women's requests for elective caesarean section in China. *Birth* publishes original research and comprehensive reviews and is a forum for debate on current issues in childbirth and education.

Midwives also use the *Journal of Advanced Nursing*, American journals such as the *Journal of Midwifery and Women's Health*, general medical journals, obstetric journals and paediatric publications to supplement their knowledge for theory and for practice.

Specialisms within nursing such as cancer nursing, services for older people, critical care and surgical nursing also have their own journals, which aim to provide more in-depth discussion about particular areas of practice. For example the August 2003 issue of *Cancer Nursing* included articles on sleep loss and depression in family care givers; the spiritual needs of patients with cancer and family caregivers; family experiences of caring for terminally patients with cancer in Hong Kong; interventions for women with newly diagnosed breast cancer; quality of life after peripheral blood stem cell transplantation; reports of drug trials and advice for healthcare providers from cancer patients. The *Journal of Psychiatric and Mental Health Nursing* aims to focus on nursing innovation and the enhanced effectiveness of nursing practice within the area of mental health nursing. Potential contributions are sent to experts for review and the focus is on a high level of scholarship. The *Journal of Advanced Nursing* aims to be an international medium for the publication of scholarly and research papers. It is available monthly on subscription only, is found in most health-care libraries and is a valuable 'heavyweight' resource for students on pre- and postregistration courses, educators and researchers.

As mentioned earlier an increasing number of journals are now produced in online formats, e.g. the *Journal of Advanced Nursing, Journal of Neonatal Nursing, Nursing Standard and Nursing Times*. The exact format differs between publications but usually includes a list of contents and abstracts from the current issues, and some archived issues. Some allow you to print off full-text articles; others require payment for this service.

There are also a growing number of online-only journals. To date these are mainly American. Some are very quirky and personal, e.g. *Nurse Beat*, which is billed as the first online journal for cardiac nurses and was set up by a nurse in the US in response to her son saying 'Mom, why don't you set up a website?' Others would seem to be using the ideal publishing medium for their content, e.g. *The Online Journal of Nursing Informatics*.

Whatever the source of the information you have collected, the following habits are recommended for purposeful and thoughtful reading.

Select one of the books or articles from your recommended reading list. As you read, ask yourself the following questions:

■ Is the author providing me with the information I need?

■ Who is writing (where do they work, what are their qualifications, do they know what they are writing about)?

■ Who is the intended audience?

■ Is the work published anywhere else?

■ Is the topic dealt with in sufficient depth?

Compare your findings with a colleague.

When reviewing the literature it is usually sensible to start with the most recent article or book first and then work backwards if more detail about original works or significant changes in thinking is required. Some authors may have written on the same topic in many different journals or books, in which case, even though you are able to access all of their publications, you should be able to extract their key thoughts on the subject by only reading one or two of them.

There is also a lot of repetition in the literature so you may find that, if you do a very detailed search, you keep coming up with essentially the same ideas. If the source you are reading does not appear to be stretching you or enabling you to get a better grasp on the subject it may not be worth reading it any further. Often it is best to restrict yourself to works that have been produced in the last 5 years. However in most subjects there are also 'classic' or 'seminal' works that need to be considered. For example, the work of Doreen Norton and others in developing a tool for the assessment of pressure sores in the 1960s was extremely significant in highlighting the importance of 'scientific' assessment in pressure area care. Similarly the work of Kurt Lewin in the 1950s on change theory has influenced much of the contemporary writings on planned organizational change. Such works are milestones in the development of our understanding about a particular subject or phenomenon.

PRIMARY AND SECONDARY SOURCES

Primary sources are articles and books written by the original authors. Secondary sources are works where the writings of others are reported on and critiqued. For example Smith P 1992 The emotional labour of nursing: its impact on interpersonal relations, management and the educational environment in nursing. Macmillan, Basingstoke is an original report into a research study carried out by the author into the nature of nursing and caring that explored how nurses care and learn to care and the effects of emotional labour on the nurses themselves and the people they care for. This book is a primary source. It has been referred to or cited in many other pieces of work, for example in Majomi et al 2003, p. 530, where it is noted that 'Smith (1992) describes care as "emotional labour", after Hochschild (1983), and argues that the demands of emotional work with people who are ill and their families are severe, but are not easily recognized or valued'.

Similarly, Taylor 2003 quotes directly from Boud et al 1985, p. 30, suggesting that reflection has the potential to recreate the totality of the practice and education experience and that: '. . .the outcomes of reflection may be a personal synthesis, integration and appropriation of knowledge, the validation of personal knowledge, a new affective state, or the decision to engage in some further action'.

Whenever direct quotes are used, i.e. the original authors' exact words are inserted into another piece of work, the full page numbers should also be supplied, as demonstrated above. This enables any reader of the secondary source to easily identify the primary source and to check for themselves whether or not the original author has been quoted correctly. Where possible it is always preferable to go to primary sources. The information is likely to be more accurate and informative than a second-hand paraphrased account or 'doctored' quote. Reviewing the original also enables you to make your own interpretations of the content and conclusions rather than relying on someone else's, which may or may not be accurate. So, after you have identified the range of references available in the area it is usually better to concentrate on primary sources.

However, if the primary sources are extremely complicated and difficult to read, it may be better to start off with a description of the original in the introductory text and then to follow it up with the original once you have some idea of the content and key issues.

SYSTEMATIC REVIEWS AND META-ANALYSES

Organizations such as the Cochrane Collaboration, the NHS Centre for Reviews and Dissemination and the Centre for Evidence-Based Nursing at the University of York suggest that, because there is currently so much health related information available to professionals, systematic reviews of this literature are required to efficiently integrate valid information and provide a basis for rational decision making. Systematic reviews use systematic methods to limit bias and reduce random errors, thus providing more reliable results from which to draw conclusions and make decisions. Meta-analysis, the use of statistical methods to summarize the results of independent studies, is thought to provide more precise estimates of the effects of health care than the results derived from individual studies.

The Cochrane Collaboration is an international organization that focuses particularly on systematic reviews of randomized controlled trials because they are likely to provide more reliable information than other sources of evidence on the differential effects of alternative forms of health care. Cochrane Reviews have a standard format. This helps readers to find the results of research quickly and to assess the validity, applicability and implications of those results. The format is also suited to electronic publication and updating, and it generates reports that are informative and readable when viewed on a computer monitor or printed.

The NHS Centre for Reviews and Dissemination is funded by the NHS Executive and the Health Departments of Scotland, Wales and Northern Ireland. It produces regular 'Effective Healthcare Bulletins' based on systematic review and synthesis of research on the clinical effectiveness and acceptability of health service interventions. This is carried out by a research team using established methodological guidelines with advice from expert consultants for each topic. Publications are available in hard copy and on line.

Before commencing any clinically focused assignment it is useful to search the websites/databases of these organizations to see whether or not they have carried out reviews in the area you are studying.

CONCLUSION

Good researching for assignments depends on taking a systematic, organized and purposeful approach to accessing relevant and appropriate resources. The key to a successful literature review is the ability to evaluate critically the work of others. You need to know what is asserted to be good practice and to be able to judge whether the arguments that are being put forward are grounded in research-based evidence and whether the research itself has been properly carried out. Evaluating the work of others is a difficult skill to learn. It involves deciding what are valid and invalid arguments, telling the difference between a good source and a bad source, seeing gaps in the literature and developing good analytical skills.

Points to remember:
- Work with your peers
- Keep a good filing system
- Take clear, relevant, appropriate notes
- Read with a purpose.

CHAPTER RESOURCES

REFERENCES

Barnes C, Mercer G 2003 Disability. Polity Press, Cambridge

Boud D, Keogh R, Walker D 1985 Reflection: turning experience into learning. Kegan Paul, London

Fader M, Clarke-O'Neill S, Cook D *et al.* 2003 Management of night-time urinary incontinence in residential settings for older people: an investigation into the effects of different pad changing regimes on skin health. Journal of Clinical Nursing 12: 374–386

Majomi P, Brown B, Crawford P 2003 Sacrificing the personal to the professional: community mental health nurses. Journal of Advanced Nursing 42: 527–538

Simons J, Reynolds J, Mannion J, Morrison L 2003 How the health visitor can help when problems between parents add to postnatal stress. Journal of Advanced Nursing 44: 400–411

Smith P 1992 The emotional labour of nursing: its impact on interpersonal relations, management and the educational environment in nursing. Macmillan, Basingstoke

Taylor C 2003 Narrating practice: reflective accounts and the textual construction of reality. Journal of Advanced Nursing 42: 244–251

Further reading

Listed below are some books on researching information, including Internet resources, that you may find useful in your studies.

Ackerman EC, Hartman K 2003 Searching and researching on the internet and world wide web, 3rd cdn. Franklin, Beedle & Associates, Wilsonville, OR

Chellen S 2000 The essential guide to the internet for health professionals. Taylor & Francis, London

Tucker DC, Craig P 2004 Pathways to nursing: a guide to library and online research in nursing and allied health. Information Today, Medford, NJ

Useful websites

British Nursing Index: http://www.bni.org.uk

Centre for Evidence Based Nursing: http://www.york.ac.uk/depts/hstd/centres/evidence/ev-intro.htm

Centre for Reviews and Dissemination: http://www.york.ac.uk/inst/crd

Cochrane Library: http://www.cochrane.org

Department of Health: http://www.dh.gov.uk/info.htm

Kings Fund: http://www.kingsfund.org.uk

Midwifery: http://midwivesonline.com
Midwives Information and Resource Service:
   http://www.midirs.org/
NHS Executive: http://www.doh.gov.uk/nhs.htm
NurseLinks: http://www.heenan.net/nurselinks/index.shtml
Nursing and healthcare resources on the web: http://www.shef.
   ac.uk/~nhcon/
Nursing Standard: http://www.nursing-standard.co.uk
Royal College of Midwifery: http://www.rcm.org.uk
Royal College of Nursing: http://www.rcn.org.uk

9 Writing skills and developing an argument

Abigail Masterson

INTRODUCTION

As students and practitioners we need to be able to communicate effectively in writing to meet the requirements of academic courses, in completing nursing and midwifery notes and care plans and to support and justify changes in practice to managers and other multi-disciplinary colleagues. Increasingly we may even wish to write for publication in order to be able to share our ideas with a wider audience. Remember that there is probably no such thing as a born writer. The successful writer is the one who regards writing as a skill to be learned, refined and constantly improved.

Writing is perhaps the most challenging part of all learning and studying. Writing involves using ideas and information to say something in a clear unambiguous way that others will understand.

Academic style is important in the development of learning skills in two ways: you will come across it in your reading and will be learning to develop it yourself through your assessed pieces of coursework. Therefore it is necessary to understand its 'rules'. Academic writing in its purest form is cautious and tentative in approach and depends on argument supported by strong evidence. The aim is to be as exact as possible and to say only what can be justified. Academic writing is designed for a very critical reader who is interested only in whether the arguments make sense and is not interested in appeals to the emotions.

Take something you have written recently, e.g. an assignment, a formal letter or minutes from a meeting. Read it through carefully and 'mark' it against the following criteria:

■ *Has all the relevant information been included?*

■ *Does it make sense?*

■ *Is it simple and to the point?*

■ *Is it legible and easy to read?*

Having marked it in this way you should be able to begin to see where some of your strengths and weaknesses are, and where it might be useful to seek further help.

DEVELOPING AN EFFECTIVE WRITING STYLE

Academic style

Although the pieces of coursework you are required to produce on your programme will probably have a variety of formats – essays, case studies, reports, critical incident analyses, reflective diaries, etc. – the principles in terms of writing style are similar. For example, in most cases it is important to justify and support the points you want to make with material that you have read. This does not mean, however, that you should cite ten authors to back up statements such as 'many women experience pain during childbirth' or 'maintaining patient/client dignity ought to be a high priority for nurses'. Make a clear distinction between what you know because you have read about it and what you know because of your own experience and reflections on those experiences.

It is vital to try and express yourself as clearly and as succinctly as possible by using short sentences and straightforward language.

Keep it simple. If you don't understand what you have written, it is unlikely that anyone else will.

For example consider this excerpt from Pearson 2003:

The concept of evidence-based practice, however, is not without controversy. The most controversial issue relates to the current focus on evidence of effectiveness. And, accordingly, the dominant approach to the systematic review of evidence favours the meta-analysis of the results of randomized controlled trials (RCTs). Indeed, the RCT is conceptualized as the 'gold standard' for evidence of effectiveness. Other quantitative methods are ranked as lower in quality in terms of the robustness of evidence. The results of interpretive and critical research are currently not regarded as producing high quality evidence. Critics of the pre-vailing privileging of the RCT and other quantitative research methods cite the arguments inherent in critiques of traditional science and in favour of the emergence of new paradigms for knowledge generation: see, for example, Fitzgerald (1995). Whilst the RCT probably is the 'best' approach for generating evidence of effectiveness, it is the case that nurses, doctors and other health professionals are concerned with much more than straightforward cause-and-effect questions. And this, rightly, is reflected in the wide range of research approaches that are utilized in the health field to generate knowledge for practice.

However clear and logical the argument, there can be a tendency to get frustrated with it very quickly if you do not agree with what the author is saying. When reading academic texts we are supposed to detach our thoughts from our feelings and put our own biases on one side in order to judge the validity of the author's arguments by their strength and soundness alone. This is practically impossible, because if we were able to do this absolutely we would not have a position from which to think about, or to judge and criticize, what we read. Eventually we may or may not decide that the author has a point but we need to give ourselves the chance to find out what is on offer and so must try not to reject opposing points of view too quickly. Instead we should use our feelings constructively by writing down our criticisms point by point.

Learning from others

A valuable aid to developing your own writing ability is to look critically at the work of others. You may find it particularly helpful to read other students' assignments and see what appears to work well and gets good marks. Similarly, when reading books and journal articles try to sort out why you prefer one author's work to another. Critically judging other people's writing in this way is a good way of increasing your understanding of what you are trying to aim for in your own writing.

Choose two journal articles that interest you. Read them thoroughly. Decide which is the better article and jot down the reasons why.

You have probably picked the article that is well structured, clear and straightforward to read.

The subject

As a student, you may be given an essay title that specifies the subject you are to write about, for example 'Clinical supervision', and may even identify the claim you are to defend or attack, for example 'Clinical supervision is a waste of scarce healthcare resources. Discuss'. However you may only be given broad guidelines: for example 'Write a 3000 word essay on a contemporary professional issue'. Your first task will therefore be to identify the subject for your essay.

How might you go about identifying a subject?

Possible sources are:

- Your own experience of clinical practice: are there issues that interest or concern you?
- Colleagues and managers: what are the current issues in your speciality, and in nursing and midwifery in general?
- Professional and specialist journals: what are the subjects being written about?

The question

The subject is the broad topic under discussion, the question is the specific issue that your argument will address. For example, given the subject 'nursing/midwifery education', you might come up with the question 'Does nursing/midwifery education contain too much theory and not enough practice?' Any subject will contain potential for lots of questions and, since you will always be writing essays, assignments and dissertations to a word limit, be it 2000 or 20000 words, the more specific you can make your question the better.

The evidence

Chapters 3, 4 and 5 looked at the practical aspects of gathering information about a subject. Having found your information, you then need to analyse it in order to see if it contains evidence that relates to either side of the question you have selected. Although you may start off with a strong hunch, or with views already well developed in one direction, it is important to keep an open mind and consider all the evidence, not just that which supports your point of view.

Structure

All written work should include an introduction where you set the context and outline the 'map' of what is to follow. This map should include what you are going to cover, why you have decided on this particular approach and how your argument will develop.

If you have been given a formal title for an assignment, such as 'Discuss the contribution of nursing/midwifery models to the development of practice', this gives some clues about what the structure and content of your essay should be. The key words in this title are 'discuss', 'nursing/midwifery models' and 'practice'. 'Discuss' highlights that there are arguments for and against and indicates that your assignment needs to consider both sides. 'Nursing/midwifery models' indicates that you need to clarify what a nursing/midwifery model is. 'Practice' means that you need to confine your discussion to the impact on practice rather than on education, research or management. The title thus can set down clear guidelines about the content that is expected.

If, however, you have just been given a topic such as 'institutionalization' you will have to decide what you think the key points and issues are. For example you might decide that you want to explore the effects of institutionalization on people with learning difficulties and put forward the case for community care in small group homes. First of all you will need to define what institutionalization is. Then discuss the contribution of people such as Erving Goffman (1968) to our understanding of this concept, identify why people with learning difficulties may become institutionalized and consider the importance of small group homes integrated into the normal social life of local communities in preventing institutionalization.

In the main body of your essay you should outline the key themes and arguments. So in our first example you might spend a paragraph defining what a nursing/midwifery model is. Then you would outline the arguments from the literature and your own experience of the advantages and disadvantages of using models in direct nursing/midwifery practice. This should take several paragraphs.

Finally you should end with a conclusion that pulls together and summarizes the key points you have made. The conclusion to the nursing/midwifery model assignment could be as follows:

Nursing models were developed mainly in the USA in the 1960s and 1970s and were associated with a desire firstly to professionalize nursing and secondly to develop a knowledge base and way of thinking that was distinct from medicine. Midwifery models have a different genesis because midwifery is less evolved as a distinct profession in the USA and therefore the UK has been at the forefront of the development of midwifery models. Nursing and midwifery models provide us with images of different ways of focusing our interventions and practices. They provide a useful structure for assessment and help nurses and midwives to make their goals of care explicit. Nevertheless, for nursing in particular, as most of the models were developed in North America they may not be readily translatable to nursing practice in the UK. Much of the language that is used – particularly in the models that derive from the USA – seems unnecessarily complicated and is very difficult to understand. The depth of assessment that is expected may not be relevant for short-stay areas such as Accident and Emergency and Day Surgery. Also, as each patient/client has different needs it may not be appropriate to use one model to plan care for all the patients or clients in one area. On balance, however, the potential associated benefits for both patients/clients and nurses of developing a focus for care that is complementary to but different from the bio-medical model is to be encouraged. Through the use and refinement of nursing and midwifery models in practice, well-structured high-quality care where the nursing/midwifery contribution becomes explicit and valued should become the norm.'

When thinking about subjects and questions, use a thought shower approach. Write down anything and everything you can think of that might be used to develop an argument. Don't be critical or selective at this stage – you could lose valuable ideas.

Using a spider diagram (demonstrated in Chapter 5), plan what you will include in one of your assignments. Make an appointment and discuss your proposed assignment with your teacher.

Each sentence in your assignment should lead logically on to the next and there should be clear signposts to your reader when you are changing subject or introducing a new point of view. Paragraphs are collections of sentences on a particular theme. When you change tack it is time for a new paragraph.

Clarity is crucial. There is often a tendency for students to use very long phrases and complicated sentences in an attempt to emulate what they read in heavyweight journals and specialist books. However, ease of reading and simplicity are far more likely to impress.

Never assume anything. Your reader has not necessarily read the same sources as you and certainly does not know what is inside your head, so you need to explain all your ideas fully and give examples to illustrate the points you are making.

The UK government is committed to ensuring that all NHS staff are information technology (IT)-literate and so the ability to word-process your work is essential. Only one side of the paper should be printed on and leave a generous space between the lines – dense text is very hard on the eyes. Spelling, punctuation and grammar do not lose you marks as such but may get in the way of the readability of your work and stop it making sense to others. If you feel that you may have a problem in these areas do seek help.

- Read the work of others. This will help you identify good and bad writing styles
- Reading helps improve vocabulary and grammar
- Practice makes perfect. Writing personal letters can help polish writing skills and boost your confidence

Compare the styles of argument and language used in the editorial columns of 'tabloid' and 'quality' (broadsheet) newspapers.

If you read something and find that you disagree with the author, think about why this is. Do you think they have got their facts wrong, or that the conclusion doesn't follow from the arguments given?

DEVELOPING AN ARGUMENT

The ability to construct an effective argument is useful in both professional and personal life. The ability to offer a reasoned argument in support of an idea or belief is central to the academic process and is a skill that you are expected to display in your written work. An essay should put forward an opinion and offer support for that opinion in the form of factual and rational evidence.

'Argument' means something very specific in its academic sense and should be distinguished from the popular use of argument to mean a verbal fight or row. An academic argument is a claim or proposition put forward, with reasons or evidence supporting it.

Why argument is important

Imagine you are in a court of law. If, at the start of the proceedings the prosecution counsel were to stand up and say: 'The defendant is guilty as charged. It's obvious, you can tell just by looking at him', it is, to say the least, unlikely that the jury would convict the defendant purely on the strength of this assertion.

What then is the missing element in the above example?

When writing an essay, just as a lawyer needs to offer evidence in support of the case for or against the defendant, you need to put forward your point of view in a structured way using evidence to persuade the reader that your point of view is the correct one.

Reflect on some situations from clinical practice where your ability to put forward a good argument might be useful.

If you were proposing to introduce a new method of patient care it is unlikely that you would be allowed to do it merely on a whim. You would need to persuade managers and medical and other health care staff of the benefits of the proposed changes, and that these outweighed any costs involved. The skills of argument are therefore of direct practical use in the clinical setting.

CASE STUDY

Domenica is the senior midwife in the midwife-led maternity unit of a community hospital. She feels that the workload of the unit is increasing and that she needs additional staff. To support her request to her manager, she gathers statistics about the numbers of births and the average length of stay, that show that the workload has been steadily increasing over the previous 18 months. On the basis of this information she requests, and is granted, permission to employ two extra part-time midwives.

Identifying an argument

In your reading as well as in your writing, it is important to be able to distinguish an argument from other types of writing.

Read the two passages below. Which is an example of an argument?

1. The nursing workforce in this hospital is stagnating. Nurses don't want to move sideways into other specialities, because they will probably have to drop a grade, and can't move up because there are no vacancies in more senior positions. Those who might want to leave the profession altogether are put off by the current economic climate and employment market.

2. The nursing workforce in this hospital is stagnating: in the year April 2002–03, among a nursing staff of 300, three F-grade posts and one G-grade post became vacant. Only one of the posts was filled by an external applicant. The figures for 2001–02 were nine F-grade posts and six G-grade posts, of which five were filled internally. Figures for the year 2000–01 were broadly similar.

Paragraph 2 is the argument, since it makes a claim (the nursing workforce is stagnating) and supports that claim with statistics from the Human Resource Department that show how the turnover of staff has slowed right down and that most posts are being filled by internal applicants.

Now read the two paragraphs again. What does paragraph I offer, given that the facts in paragraph 2 are correct?

Paragraph 1 offers an explanation for the facts given in paragraph 2. It seems, on the face of it, a reasonable explanation, but it is worth remembering that for any one set of circumstances there may be more than one explanation.

If you were the manager of the hospital in the example above, what could you do to test the truth of the explanation offered for the slow-down in staff movement?

One possible way would be to carry out a survey of the staff and see if the reasons they give for reluctance to move tally with those suggested.

A police officer arrives at a road junction and finds two dented cars and two angry drivers. The officer has no way of knowing who is at fault without looking at the physical evidence and taking statements from the drivers and any witnesses. Sometimes one explanation will seem more plausible than another, but this does not necessarily make it the correct one.

Description of facts and opinions is a necessary part of any argument: in fact it is impossible to argue without describing various aspects of the subject you are arguing about. However, it is quite possible to describe without arguing. Take away the statement 'The nursing workforce in this hospital is stagnating' in the second paragraph above and all that is left is a collection of statistics.

When you present information that is relevant to the argument you are making, you must tell your reader or your listener why you are doing so and how you are using the facts.

Fact and opinion

When you are collecting the evidence that you will use to support your argument you must be careful to distinguish between objective facts and opinions.

In the passage below, what is fact and what opinion?

There are 644 000 nurses, midwives and health visitors in the UK and most of them have suffered from stress as a direct result of their work.

The number of registered nurses, midwives and health visitors in the UK is something that could be established with reasonable accuracy from published figures, and is therefore fact: whether the majority have suffered from work-related stress is more open to debate, however self-evident it appears. If you were to include a paragraph like this in an essay you would either have to qualify your statement or provide evidence to support the opinion (the results of a survey, for example).

When preparing an argument, think of yourself as a lawyer getting ready for a court case and ask yourself:

■ What is the charge? (i.e. what is the subject of the essay or discussion?)

■ Am I prosecuting or defending? (i.e. what is the claim I am making)?

■ What evidence do I have that supports my case and will convince the jury that the defendant is innocent (or guilty)?

Let's look at some of the methods that are often used in place of reasoned arguments. In each of the examples below, try to identify where these fail. Remember the definition of argument given at the start of the chapter when you are thinking about this.

Example 1
We should bring back capital punishment: murder is a dreadful crime and murderers should pay the ultimate penalty for it.

A list of claims, eloquently made, can be very persuasive (politicians are generally very good at this) but it does not constitute an argument, because there is no inference or chain of reasoning.

Look again at the above example: try crossing out any one of the statements. Does it make any difference to the other two?

It seems to make no difference: any one of the claims might be true or false, without affecting the truth or falsity of any of the other claims. This is therefore an unsupported assertion.

Example 2
'If you don't stop teasing your brother, I will send you to your room.' (Parent to child)

Midwives who do not accept the new working practices will be deemed to be in breach of their contract of employment and subject to immediate dismissal. (Hospital notice)

St Ignatius Hospital – the home of the truly professional nurse. (Recruitment advertisement)

The first two statements use the threat of harm of some kind, the third, promise of reward. Threats and seduction use physical or psychological coercion to cause a person to act in a particular way or adopt a certain point of view.

Consider your reaction to the following paragraphs. What factors might affect your reactions in each case?

Example 3
The wholesale slaughter of helpless creatures in these animal Belsens, a direct result of this unnatural craving for flesh, represents an unjustifiable oppression of sentient beings.

Demand for increased quantities of meat has led to intensive 'factory farming' methods, where the welfare of livestock may take second place to economics.

The rights and wrongs of farming and animal welfare are outside the scope of this book: our interest here is the language used. In the first paragraph the language is strong, emotive, even violent: there is little doubt here what the author's views are on the subject. The second paragraph is more measured: it could be read as either neutral, or perhaps slightly favourable – your own views on the subject might affect your opinion here.

Emotive language has its place but should not be used as a substitute for reasoned argument. It is unlikely to persuade those who do not already share your point of view and it may actually put off those who are neutral on the issue.

Are these reasonable claims? If not, what is the problem with them?

Example 4
All midwives know that tried and trusted methods are preferable to constant change.
    Midwives are constantly being asked to take on aspects of the medical role.

In both cases, the question must be: How do you know? Have you actually asked any midwives? If so how many, where and when?

Therefore avoid rash, universal statements in your writing such as 'Everybody knows that. . .'.

Consider also: even if everybody does believe something, and you can prove that they believe it, does that necessarily mean that it is true? After all, 600 years ago, most people believed that the world was flat and that the Earth was the centre of the universe. (On the other hand, beware the modernist assumption that any beliefs and opinions held by our ancestors are automatically wrong.)

Read the following statements: how does the writer attempt to persuade you to their point of view?

Example 5
Surely it must be acknowledged that many people abuse the welfare system.
    It is perfectly obvious that nurses have a role in the operating department.

Did you notice the way in which the words 'surely' and 'perfectly obvious' are used? These are persuader words and involve a kind of false logic – the 'Emperor's new clothes' argument. This refers to the classic story by Hans Christian Anderson in which two tailors deceive the emperor and most of his subjects by claiming that they are weaving a marvellous cloth that can only be seen by the very wise. In fact they work at an empty loom and weave nothing but, since nobody likes to be thought unwise, everybody claims to be able to see the cloth and in the end it takes the innocent wisdom of a child to break the self-deception that all the adults have succumbed to.

There are various other types of surrogate argument, but those outlined above are the most common and you should avoid them in your writing. Always ask yourself of any statement that you read or hear 'Why should I believe this to be true?'

HOW ARGUMENTS WORK

We have just considered some of the substitutes for rational argument that you may encounter in your reading. Sometimes these are easy to spot but they can also be well concealed. In these cases it can be helpful to break the argument down and examine it more closely. In doing this, you can also begin to see how arguments work and how to go about constructing your own.

Read the passage below. Can you spot any flaws in the argument? (If you are not familiar with the two studies cited, accept for the purposes of the exercise that they do demonstrate what the paragraph claims that they do. Pre-operative visiting is the term used for a system in which a theatre nurse sees surgical patients on the ward the afternoon or evening before surgery. During the visit they are given the opportunity to discuss what will happen to them – what they will see, hear, feel, where they will be when they wake up etc. – and to ask questions.)

Example 6

Classic studies by Boore (1975) and Hayward (1975) demonstrated that, if patients receive information about their treatment in advance, they recover more quickly, require less analgesia and are discharged earlier than those who do not receive this information. The information could be conveyed by means of a preoperative visit from a member of the theatre team, who because of their specialist knowledge is well placed to describe what the patient will experience and answer any questions. Preoperative visiting therefore would bring benefits to the patient, and it is theatre nurses who should be carrying out such visits.

First establish what the subject of the discussion is. In this case, it is preoperative visiting by nurses who work in the operating department.

The next thing to establish is the position which the author appears to take up, the claim which is to be defended. Sometimes this is obvious, at other times less so, but you need to be clear about the claim made before you can judge the quality of the evidence provided in support.

What is the claim made in the passage above?

The author actually appears to make two claims, firstly that 'pre-operative visiting... would bring benefits to the patient' and secondly that 'theatre nurses should [carry out preoperative visits]'. This is a mistake in itself: claims should be made singly, not bunched together. Claims need to be supported in some way.

What is the evidence presented in support of each claim?

Let's consider the first claim, that preoperative visiting benefits the patient. The author starts by citing two research studies that have demonstrated benefits to patients from preoperative information giving: the first sentence thus offers facts, the accuracy of which may be easily checked. The second sentence then puts forward a suggestion, namely that theatre staff could give this information during a preoperative visit. It therefore seems reasonable to conclude that, on the face of it, patients will benefit from preoperative visits.

Note, however, that this makes the presumption that patients prefer on the whole to recover quickly and have short stays in hospital. Watch out for this kind of presumption and ask yourself 'is it reasonable to presume this?' For example the argument that: 'regular exercise makes you fit, slim and healthy: everybody should exercise' presumes that everybody wants to be these things: is this the case?

Let's turn to the second claim, that theatre nurses should be doing preoperative visits. Here the support offered for the claim is less obvious, but seems to be that theatre nurses have specialist knowledge. The chain of inference is therefore:

Patients need information (because it improves the outcome of surgery)

↓

Theatre nurses have the information (because they are specialists with specialist knowledge)

↓

Preoperative visits are a means of passing on this information

↓

Theatre nurses should do preoperative visits

There are, however, a number of presumptions here. Can you spot what they are?

First, is it reasonable to claim that theatre nurses have specialist knowledge? Some might well do, but not all. It might be better to say 'an experienced member of the theatre team' or 'a specially trained member of the team'. Second, is the theatre nurse well placed to answer any questions? How about those that relate to the proposed surgery, or the anaesthetic to be used? Third, is a preoperative visit necessarily the best way of conveying the information that the patient might need?

Does the conclusion therefore follow from the evidence put forward? Should we accept that theatre nurses should be the ones to provide information? It would be perfectly possible to argue that ward-based nurses have more opportunity to develop the necessary rapport than a theatre nurse during a brief visit.

There is one final point to note, and that is the way in which the two claims, i.e. (1) that patients would benefit from preoperative visits and (2) that theatre nurses should do preoperative visits, are put together at the end in a way that suggests that the one implies the other when they are, as we have seen, two separate ideas. This is called conflation.

CONSIDERING THE EVIDENCE

Evidence may take various forms. The simplest, most direct form is fact.

- 'There are approximately 644000 practitioners registered with the Nursing and Midwifery Council'
- 'The functions of the Nursing and Midwifery Council are enshrined in the Nursing and Midwifery Order 2001 of the UK Parliament'.

Both these facts could be checked and verified.

Certain value statements are also admissible evidence in argument:

- 'Human life is intrinsically valuable'
- 'Nursing is a caring profession'.

Neither of these statements could be proven objectively but both express ideas that are almost universal and could thus be used to support an argument. (This is not the same as the mistaken universal belief about the flatness of the world mentioned earlier in the chapter, because this was later disproved by observation and experiment. No scientific enquiry could prove or disprove either of the above statements.)

The third form of evidence is opinion. Opinion is not a prejudice or an unconsidered point of view but is arrived at by a logical thought process. An argument consists of a claim (the conclusion), supported by evidence (the premise or premises). By convention, the premises are given first, followed by the conclusion:

- *Premise 1*: To intentionally kill an innocent human being is both illegal and immoral in all cultures

- *Premise 2*: Active euthanasia involves the intentional killing of another human being by lethal injection or other means

- *Conclusion*: Active euthanasia is therefore morally wrong.

The conclusion, that euthanasia is morally wrong, could then be used to support an argument in favour of greater efforts to improve palliative care.

Included in this type of evidence may be the expert opinions of specialists in the topic under discussion: these usually come from books and journal articles. If you quote from these, you must remember to acknowledge your sources, using an accepted reference and citation system (see Chapter 8 for more details).

Note that this kind of argument is never completely watertight: you can pick holes in any argument you come across, but this doesn't matter. One of the things that an essay tests is your ability to marshal facts in support of an argument.

STRUCTURING THE ARGUMENT

Like a lawyer in court, your task in an essay is to convince the jury (your reader) that your point of view is the correct one (or at least, one that is worth considering). As the lawyer uses evidence and statements by witnesses to build up the case, so you have to show how your evidence supports your argument.

The above example demonstrates one basic argument that could be used against euthanasia but is open to attack by anyone who believes that there is a moral distinction between murder as such and the use of active methods to kill the terminally ill. As a general rule it is a good idea to defend your overall argument (that active euthanasia should not be permitted) with as many supporting arguments as you can develop in the time and space allowed.

What other arguments could be used to support the view that active euthanasia should not be permitted?

You could approach the argument as follows:

- *Premise*: The deliberate taking of life is wrong
- *Supporting evidence*: The law and customs of all cultures, the intrinsic value of human life
- *Premise*: The possibility of euthanasia would undermine the basic relationship of trust and confidence that should exist between patient and nurse or doctor
- *Supporting evidence*: Medical and nursing ethical codes, Hippocratic oath, statements by professional bodies
- *Premise*: The availability of euthanasia would reduce the drive to improve standards of palliative care
- *Supporting evidence*: Expert testimony, publications by specialists in palliative care
- *Premise*: It would be impossible to legislate effectively and safely for euthanasia
- *Supporting evidence*: The history of attempts to legislate, the impossibility of legislating to cover all circumstances, analogy with misuse of other laws and their extension in ways not envisaged by their creators
- *Conclusion*: Active euthanasia should not be permitted.

Note how each of the premises that support the main conclusion are in a sense the conclusions of supporting arguments.

HOW ARGUMENTS GO WRONG

An argument can go wrong: either because the premises are faulty and therefore the conclusion does not follow or because the premises are true, but do not support the conclusion.

What is wrong with the argument below?

All midwives are female.

Chris is a midwife.

Therefore Chris is female.

It can be easily shown that some midwives are male, therefore the first premise is untrue and the conclusion does not follow. Note, however, that the form of the argument is perfectly valid. If all midwives were indeed female, then the conclusion would be true.

What is wrong with this argument?

All midwives are female.

Chris is female.

Therefore Chris is a midwife.

In this case the problem is with the form of the argument. Even if it were true that all midwives are female, and that Chris is female, it does not follow that Chris is a midwife: she might be an engineer, or an airline pilot, or anything else. She might even be a midwife, but this argument doesn't prove it.

Consider the following statements/arguments, and try to identify the problems with them. The important thing is to be able to spot when and where an argument is going wrong.

1. Mr Lister married his sister.

2. You will meet a dark stranger and your financial affairs will be affected.

These statements are ambiguous: in (1) the word 'sister' can be understood in several different ways, as can the word 'married': did Mr Lister marry his biological sister and commit incest? Was Mr Lister the clergyman who officiated at his sister's wedding? (In fact, neither interpretation is correct. Joseph Lister, an eminent Victorian surgeon, married his theatre sister, in the best traditions of nurse–doctor romances!) In example (2), which might be found in the horoscope pages of a magazine, the whole statement could mean any number of different things.

3. Eight out of ten cats prefer Kat Din.

Here it is the information that is not supplied that is crucial. The statement sounds like the results of an experiment, but how many cats were involved? 10? 100? 10 000? What were they offered as an alternative to Kat Din?

4. The argument for the use of corporal punishment as a legitimate educational tool is supported by the works of many famous authors such as Charles Dickens, and also by several prominent politicians.

You may have wondered what special knowledge of education the people referred to possess. Certainly, they are well known, even famous, but are they qualified to comment on the subject of corporal punishment and its effectiveness as a teaching tool?

Using authorities is acceptable, but only to lend support in their area of expertise.

5. Nurses and doctors are always going on about the dangers of smoking, but lots of them smoke, so it can't be that bad for you.

In this kind of fallacy the argument is directed against the failings of individuals in order to discredit the argument put forward. However, in the example above, does the behaviour of some health professionals discredit the idea that smoking is bad for you, or does it simply illustrate that human beings are fallible, and don't always live up to the ideals they express.

6. I submit, ladies and gentlemen of the jury, that the witness is lying when he says he saw the defendant breaking into the house. The witness is known to have a grudge against the defendant, and has also lied to the police in the past when accused of a motoring offence.

7. It's not worth treating these people. They don't listen to advice and they won't alter their diet or their exercise habits.

These examples illustrate the same fallacy as statement 5. The problem is that there may be occasions when it seems acceptable to direct attention to the failings of an individual. Example 7 illustrates one aspect of a debate that is beginning to be heard more often nowadays. What do you think? (And why?)

8. The majority of midwives are confident that doctors regard them as fellow professionals.

We saw an example of this fallacy, the appeal to popular belief, in Example 4 above. The fact that a majority believes something to be true does not necessarily mean that it is true (although, of course, it may be). For this reason, the results of opinion polls on contentious issues should be treated with some caution.

9. I believe God exists: it has not been proved God does not exist, therefore God exists.

10. I've never known using egg white and oxygen on pressure sores to do any harm, so it must be doing some good.

This is the appeal to ignorance, arguing that, because we don't know something is not true, it *is* true.

11. Fred Bloggs always tells the truth.

How do you know?

Fred Bloggs told me so.

How do you know he wasn't lying?

Because he always tells the truth.

This is the circular argument: the conclusion of the argument, that Fred Bloggs tells the truth, is used as one of the premises that supports the conclusion. You may have encountered it in your work in this form:

Why do we do 'it' (e.g. changing a dressing, dealing with patients/clients, organizing the off-duty rota) this way?

Because we've always done it this way.

But why have we always done it this way?

Because we always have.

12. People who drive red cars have more accidents than those who drive cars of another colour. Therefore if no cars were coloured red, there would be fewer accidents.

This is a non sequitur (Latin, 'it does not follow'). The argument suggests that it is the colour of the car that causes the accident, not the behaviour of the person driving it!

GETTING STARTED

Most of the hard work should be done by now – you have collected your resources together and organized your thoughts. Your work does not have to be perfect. Students sometimes miss submission dates or do not start writing at all because of an unrealistic desire for perfection. Practice is important but two or three drafts of any piece of work should be sufficient. Try not to write and edit at the same time otherwise you may lose your capacity to think clearly as you get bogged down in the intricacies of spelling and grammar. Particularly when working on personal computers there is a great temptation and potential for wasting time by spellchecking practically every sentence and perpetually checking the word count.

- If you are working for a whole day, spend the morning writing and the afternoon editing
- If you are working for part of the day, write for a couple of hours and edit for an hour

Nothing is more off-putting than a blank page and, if you cannot think of a punchy opening sentence or introductory paragraph, start somewhere in the middle and work backwards. Do not try and complete your task in one go. The task will feel enormous and impossible that way. Break the job down into manageable stages. If you get stuck at one bit try another part and then go back to the first one once you have freed up your thoughts. Finally, it is important to trust your impressions and to have faith in yourself. There is usually no such thing as one right answer. You need to work out what your own thoughts are on the area. It is important to have your own opinion but it must be based on reasonable evidence rather than gut feeling or prejudice. Do not be constrained by fear of looking a fool or getting it wrong – have a go.

Prior to submitting a completed piece of work check the following:
1. Is the right question/title at the head of your work?
2. Have you included all the relevant personal details, e.g.
    - Your name
    - Candidate/examination number
    - Course name
    - Lecturer's/marker's name?
3. Is your work legible and ordered:
    - Printed in an appropriate font size and type
    - Only one side of the paper used
    - Organized logically
    - Pages numbered?
4. Is the spelling and punctuation accurate?
    - Use spell checkers and dictionaries to help but remember that they will not pick up errors such as the misuse of 'their' and 'there', etc.
5. Have you kept a back-up copy on a disk in case the original is inadvertently lost or there is a problem with your computer?

Handing in your work and receiving a mark and/or comments is not the end of the process. If you want to progress and improve it is important to note the comments made by the marker and try to make constructive use of their feedback.

ACCEPTING FEEDBACK

One of the most useful ways of developing yourself, both as a student and as a practitioner, is the ability to listen to others and to make the most of constructive criticism. You will receive feedback in practice placements, after doing presentations in class and on assignments. As I suggested in the introduction, there is no such thing as a born writer: practice is essential. Often we tend to compare our efforts with those of experienced writers rather than our peers and to get very disillusioned as a result. It is important to take every opportunity you are offered for feedback and to try and learn from the feedback you are given, however painful this feels at first. It is always hard when you have spent a lot of time and energy on something not to get the mark you hoped for or to receive pages and pages of criticism back from your lecturer or the editor of a journal. It is important to try and take such feedback as part of your development as a writer rather than as a criticism of you as an individual or a practitioner.

Nobody likes receiving negative comments about their work, particularly if they result in referral or failure of part of a course. When such things happen we often tend to try to blame others: the paper was hard, the marker didn't like us, the lecturer/our off-duty didn't give us sufficient time to revise. However in order to grow and develop we need to acknowledge our own mistakes and take responsibility for our own performance. You may wish to turn to Chapter 2 for further discussion of the importance of taking responsibility for your own learning and development.

If you get a mark that you are not happy with or are referred on a piece of coursework, do not go and see your lecturer immediately. Give yourself time to adjust and get over the feelings of sadness, anger and disappointment. When you do go to see your lecturer, take along your assignment and any comments from the marker. The comments can act as a guide for the tutorial and can be useful prompts and pointers if you are required to re-write the assignment.

I always keep a copy of the first essay I ever wrote for an academic course. If I ever feel disenchanted by feedback, I can read through and remind myself how my style and competence have developed.

CONCLUSION

In this chapter we have explored the process of writing an assignment. You have been encouraged to be critical about what you read and the importance of clarity and structure in your preparation and your writing has been emphasized. In written work and discussion you need to be able to put forward your point of view clearly and effectively. This means telling your reader/audience exactly what the point you are making is, what evidence you are using in support and how that evidence supports what you are saying. Arguments go wrong either because the evidence is untrue or because it does not support the conclusion. Successful writing, as with so many other things in life, perfectly illustrates the truth of the old adage 'practice makes perfect'.

- Answer the question
- The aim of an argument is to get the other person to accept that your point of view is the correct one, or is at least worth considering
- When you argue, you must support your claims with evidence
- The evidence must be true, clearly stated and relevant to the argument
- Avoid substitutes for argument
- Succinct, straightforward, structured writing is the ideal
- Use feedback positively to help you refine your skills

CHAPTER RESOURCES

REFERENCES

Boore J 1976 An investigation into the effects of some aspects of pre-operative preparation on post-operative stress and recovery. Thesis, RCN Steinbeck Collection, London

Goffman E 1968 Asylums. Penguin Books, Harmondsworth

Hayward J 1975 Information: a prescription against pain. Royal College of Nursing, London

Pearson A 2003 Guest editorial: liberating our conceptualisation of 'evidence'. Journal of Advanced Nursing 44: 441–442

Further reading

Barrass R 2003 Students must write: a guide to better writing in coursework and examinations. Routledge, London

Race P 2003 How to study: practical tips for university students. Blackwell, Oxford

Williams D 2003 Writing skills in practice: a practical guide for health professionals. Jessica Kingsley, London

10 Presentation of written material

Sian Maslin-Prothero

INTRODUCTION

The aim of this chapter is to assist you in preparing and presenting material either for oral or written presentations. The first part of the chapter looks at different styles of writing and the remainder looks at the presentation of written material. This will provide you with a framework, which you can adapt to meet your requirements.

Being asked to write something, be it an essay, a report or an article, can be a daunting task. If you are undertaking any course of study, completing a written assignment is still the most common form of assessing student learning. How to write an essay has been covered in Chapters 8 and 9; this chapter will examine other ways of presenting written material.

You will already have considerable experience of writing and presenting material for others, for example completing assignments as part of course work in school or college or, in practice areas, writing care plans and reports to colleagues in handover or ward rounds.

In each of these scenarios you have to identify what is the most important information, i.e. what needs to be communicated, and what is not essential. You then provide the essential information in the most appropriate format and style. This will be different according to whether you are providing a presentation (to an audience) or a written piece of work.

DIFFERENT STYLES OF WRITING

In Chapter 9 you looked at writing skills and developing an argument. There may be other forms of writing you may have to do as part of your course or as a daily activity. These will include some of the following:

- Letters to friends and family
- Job and course applications
- Lecture notes
- Reports on patients and clients
- Projects
- Memos
- Essays
- Examinations
- Reviews on books or articles.

Each one of the above has special features that need to be considered prior to preparation and before actually writing.

- *What is the material for?*
- *Who is going to read it?*
- *How long should it be?*
- *Should it be written in the first person or third person?*

WRITING FOR DIFFERENT PURPOSES

The style and content you adopt for writing will vary depending on the task. A letter to a member of your family or to a friend is likely to be very different from a memo sent to a colleague.

BOX 10.1	*Personal letter*

Dear Pat

How are you? I haven't heard from you since you moved into your new house.

I hope the move went well. It must be a real luxury having a fridge – not having to leave your milk and butter outside the back door!

Have you been climbing recently? Charlotte and I have been to the indoor climbing centre in Nottingham – it is so small in comparison to Bristol's. The centre is a long way from where we live and, unfortunately, there is no direct bus. The thought of trying to find a climbing partner is a bit daunting – I had got so used to climbing with you and Kym.

My new job is going well. People have been really welcoming. Last night we were all invited round to a colleague's house for supper. They have children the same age as Jack and Charlotte. Fortunately, the children seemed to get on well. Both Paul and the children are settling into their new environment.

Do write soon and let me know how things are going with you. Send my love to Chris.

Love from

Sian

The style of a personal letter is often less formal and more familiar. In comparison, a memorandum to a colleague will be different (Fig. 10.1).

FIGURE 10.1   *An office memorandum*

MEMORANDUM

To: Sian Maslin-Prothero
             Lecturer

From: Rachel Clarke
             Head of Department

Re: Transferable skills in full-time
             degree programmes

Date: 23 November 2000

Thank you for your letter of 21 November 2000. Would you please let me have a paper briefly outlining how transferable skills have already been incorporated into the existing programmes, and any personal developments?

HOW TO PREPARE A PROJECT

You are likely to have to undertake a project as part of a course or in your work environment. This can seem a frightening prospect, although it can also be a satisfying experience. The key to success is preparation; this involves developing a plan. Before embarking on this you need to consider the following questions:

What have I got to do?

Use the assignment guidelines to help you decide:

- the subject
- the word limit
- the date for submission.

How much time do I have to complete the project?

Be realistic. You need to structure and plan your time. Remember to include some extra time to allow for events such as lost data or computer breakdown. Once you have drawn up a timetable, try to stick to it.

Drawing on Chapter 1, which discussed planning and organizing your time, completing a project is similar to writing an essay (see Chapters 8 and 9). The flow diagram shown in Figure 10.2 can help you organize your work effectively. Your aims and objectives (see Chapter 1 for definition) will be the basis for deciding what information you require in order to complete the project.

HOW TO PREPARE A REPORT

The structure of a report is different from an essay or a letter. Reports are written because there is a need for specific information: for instance where a problem has been identified and requires investigation. Reports are written for a purpose and target a specific audience. They are statements presented in a logical sequence leading to conclusions and possible recommendations for future action. A good report is characterized by its objectivity and systematic presentation. Reports have a format that leads the reader quickly to the main themes and findings.

Content of a report

All information contained in the report must be relevant, concise and substantiated, and it must be presented in a clear, logical sequence.

FIGURE 10.2	*Planning and implementing project work*

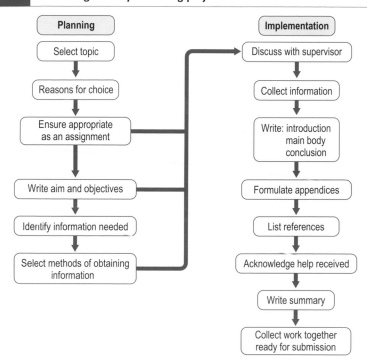

The report should have an introduction in which the terms of reference are defined. The terms of reference include: who has commissioned the report; why they have asked for the report to be written; the purpose of the report; who the report is for; and who is going to read the final report. Essential background material may be included, or you can put details in the appendices. Some or all of the following may be included in the report:

- The **method** is where you tell the reader how you went about obtaining the information or analysed the information for the report
- The **results** are where you present your findings
- The **discussion** is where you discuss the implications of your findings
- The **summary** is where you summarize the results
- The **recommendations** are based on your findings.

The writing style should be clear and specific. Aim to use short and simple sentences, so that the reader easily understands the report. The report should be coherent and non-anecdotal. All sections, subsections and points must have headings and must be numbered and indented.

This is so that the report flows logically and information can be easily retrieved. Box 10.2 illustrates the layout of a report.

BOX 10.2	*Report*

Abstract
1. Introduction
   1.1 Style
      1.1.1 Ensure that the writing style; language and level are appropriate for the intended audience.
   1.2 Report writing is formal; reports are usually written in the third person.
   1.3 Who am I writing for?
   1.4 What is their knowledge of the subject?
2. Structure
   2.1 Reports often need to be read quickly, so ensure that the reader can find their way around the document easily.
      2.1.1 Sections and subsections should be numbered appropriately.
   2.2 Your introduction places the report in context. The conclusion draws the argument together and makes recommendations where appropriate.
   2.3 The abstract should be a precis of the introduction and conclusion.
3. Material
   3.1 Be selective and stick to the point.
   3.2 Report writing is a review of all the evidence, not a personal view.
   3.3 Start with the most important things first, then add the necessary detail.
   3.4 Avoid repeating yourself. You may find you need to reorder the material.
4. Conclusion
   4.1 Use clear, simple language and stick to the point. Break the report into sections and subsections, with headings to guide the reader.
   4.2 Number the pages.
   4.3 If there is a specific word length, stick to it.

Your report will need an abstract, an introduction, the main body, a conclusion, recommendations and appendices. Any diagrams must be appropriate, numbered and clearly labelled. Only include diagrams if they are relevant and referred to in the report, otherwise there is no point in including them. If you have a word processing package, look under the 'Help' section; most packages have a system for report writing.

To summarize, to achieve effective communication you should use clear, simple language with well-laid-out sections and appropriate use of headings and summaries that will guide the reader through the report.

REVIEWING A BOOK OR ARTICLE

The ability to critically evaluate the work of others is important for a number of reasons: preparation for any assignment or project necessitates the individual critically evaluating the work of others in the area – not all research or reports have been reviewed by referees or peers. Critical evaluation is about being able to evaluate other people's work, both positively and negatively, thus judging the quality of the work. This is a valuable and useful skill to develop, and should be used when you read papers, reports and books (see Chapters 8 and 9).

You may be asked to review a published book either as part of your course or for a journal. You will be provided with specific guidelines on what is expected in the review. This usually includes:

- a specified word limit for the review
- details of the book to be reviewed, e.g. author(s), title, place of publication, publisher, date of publication, number of pages, ISBN number and the price of the book.

The review is expected to provide a clear idea of the content of the book, and should be an interesting and critical appraisal of the work and its place in the existing literature, as well as providing an insight to current thinking and trends in nursing. For further information on writing a book review see Johnson (1995) and Watson (1998, 1999).

NON-DISCRIMINATORY LANGUAGE

The aim of language is to communicate. Our use of language reflects our own attitudes. Therefore, if the language we use leads to misunderstanding or offends individuals, we will experience problems with communicating.

When using language, whether written or the spoken word, you need to be sure that you are not excluding people or discriminating against them. The way we speak and the language we use can reinforce inaccurate stereotypes. For example, the term 'mother and toddler group' insinuates that only mothers are responsible for childcare, and this is not the case. The term playgroup actually describes what is available and includes all carers.

Non-sexist language

The term 'man' should not be used to refer to both sexes. There are non-sexist alternatives (Table 10.1).

- He/him/his are not universal terms for men and women
- Very few occupations or roles are exclusive to either males or females – the language used should reflect the job or task being performed

TABLE 10.1	*Sexist and non-sexist terminology*
Sexist	**Non-sexist**
Mankind	People, humanity
Manpower	Workforce
Forefathers	Ancestors
Fireman	Firefighter
Headmaster	Headteacher

The most important thing is to think, and to avoid discriminatory language in your written and spoken words. This is most likely to occur when using pronouns. A pronoun is a word used instead of a proper or other noun to indicate a person or thing already mentioned. For example: I, me, she, her, he, him, it, you, they, them, are all pronouns.

There are several ways to avoid discriminatory language.

- Avoid the pronoun altogether – use 'a', 'an', 'the' instead. For example: 'A nurse has his special patient' could be written: 'A nurse has a special patient' or 'All nurses have their special patients'
- Use 'they': 'Once a nurse has registered to practice he knows in what area he wants to work' could be written: 'Once a nurse has registered to practice they know in what area they want to work'
- Use both pronouns 'he/she' or 'his/her': For example: 'A nurse has her/his special patient'. However, this can be clumsy
- Use a second-person pronoun, 'you': 'As a nurse, you have your special patient'
- Use the first person plural, 'we': 'We nurses have our special patients'
- Use 'one' (with caution, as it also has class connotations): 'As a nurse, one has a special patient'
- Use a plural pronoun with a singular antecedent (e.g. everyone, every, etc.): 'Every nurse has their special patient' or 'Everyone has their special patient'

Remember . . . think before you write or speak.

The use of non-discriminatory language might seem difficult but, with practice, it becomes natural to use terms that do not discriminate against people because of their gender, sexuality, race, etc.

COPYRIGHT AND PLAGIARISM

It is unclear how frequently plagiarism occurs but the aim is often to deceive, so many cases go undetected. It is important that you reference all material used. If you include other people's ideas or work without acknowledging their contribution then you are plagiarising and risk failing your course or losing your job (see Chapter 5). People plagiarise for different reasons: ignorantly, innocently and deliberately.

If you copy a quotation from a book or article, you must credit the author, i.e. reference their work including name, date of publication and page number. Referencing other people's work is very important for a number of reasons: it enables the reader to refer to the original work and check the authenticity of the quotation if they wish to; it enables the reader to use the source for their own research; and it helps the reader to distinguish between other people's ideas and your own. The safest way of avoiding plagiarism is to acknowledge the sources you have used. When preparing an assignment make notes using the following 'Avoiding plagiarism' guide.

Avoiding plagiarism

■ Separate direct quotations from your own work by using quotation marks
■ Always cite the precise source in your reference list
■ List all sources used in the bibliography
■ When paraphrasing another's work, identify the original source, including the author and date of publication

You may refer to another person's work by paraphrasing in your own words. In this situation you must still reference the original work using the author and date. This is referred to as the primary source. In the case where an author you are reading refers to another author and their work, and you do not access the original work, you may cite this work. This is sometimes referred to as secondary source, for example 'Brown (1978, cited in Maslin-Prothero 1994)'.

To successfully avoid the pitfall of plagiarism consider the following points:

■ Don't attempt the question until you understand it
■ Do consult your lecturer and colleagues
■ Plan your time carefully
■ Reference your notes and sources as you go along. Don't wait until you have completed the essay and then try to remember where they came from

REFERENCE AND CITATION SYSTEMS

It is an essential requirement when researching and producing a written project that all sources used are properly acknowledged. It is important that you employ and become used to a standardized reference system.

These guidelines describe the Harvard and the Vancouver systems of referencing, which are the most commonly used. You may use another system, but bear in mind that it is important to keep to a standard form throughout your written contribution.

BOX 10.3   *Definitions*

- **Reference**: a bibliographic description including author(s), date, title, publisher and place of publication
- **Reference list**: a bibliographic list of items referred to in the text
- **Bibliography**: a list of other relevant material used but not referred to in the text
- **Annotated bibliography**: a bibliography where each reference is accompanied by a critical or explanatory note

---

The Harvard system of referencing

The box below shows how to cite a reference in the text and create an alphabetically complied list of references at the end of the text.

BOX 10.4

Doctors who make the diagnosis are in a powerful position. Access to such power is controlled by professional associations with their own vested interests to protect (Naidoo and Wills 1994). The 1858 Medical Act established the General Medical Council which was authorized to regulate doctors, oversee medical education and keep a register of qualified practitioners (Hart 1994).

Medical colleges resisted the entry of women to the profession for many years. In 1901 there were 36 000 medical practitioners, of whom 212 were women. There is evidence that Black and Asian doctors face discrimination in their medical careers (Tschudin 1994a). This implies that ability is not the sole criterion for gaining a place to train in medicine or in subsequent career progression. Special counselling is a good idea in such cases (Tschudin 1994b).

References
Hart, C. (1994) *Behind the mask: nurses, their unions and nursing policy.* Baillière Tindall, London
Naidoo, J. and Wills, J. (1994) *Health promotion: foundation for practice.* Baillière Tindall, London
Tschudin, V. (1994a) *Deciding ethically: a practical approach to nursing challenges.* Baillière Tindall, London
Tschudin, V. (1994b) *Counselling.* Baillière Tindall, London

---

At every point where the text refers to a particular document, insert the author(s) last name, first name initial(s) and year of publication. Use lower case letters after the year if referring to more than one piece of work published in the same year by the same author.

Book references

Give the following facts, in this order:

- Name of the author(s), editor(s) or the institution responsible for writing the book
- Year of publication in brackets
- Title and subtitle, underlined (or in italic type)
- Volume and individual issue number (if any)
- Edition, if not the first
- Publisher
- Place of publication, if known.

BOX 10.5   Doyal, L. (ed.) (1998) *Women and health services.* Open University Press, Buckingham

---

Journal references

A reference to an article in a journal contains the following information, in the order listed below:

- Author(s)
- Year of publication in brackets
- Title of article
- Title of journal (in italic type)
- Volume number
- Issue number in brackets
- Specific date (for a weekly journal)
- Inclusive pages.

BOX 10.6   Watson, R. (1999) Another message from the book reviews editor. *Journal of Advanced Nursing* 29(6), 1283–1284

References to contributions in books

Enter under the name of contributing author and include the relevant page numbers.

BOX 10.7   Martindale, K. (2001) Getting the most from reading and lectures. In: Maslin-Prothero, S. E. (ed.) (2001) *Baillière's study skills for nurses,* 2nd edn. Baillière Tindall, London, ch. 5, pp. 97–109

Handbooks, directories in single or several volumes

BOX 10.8	Cambridge Information and Research Services Limited (1986) Industrial Development Guide 1986, 8th edn. Longman, Harlow

Theses and dissertations

Include the details of level and awarding institution.

BOX 10.9	Owen, S. (1999) A pluralistic evaluation of services for women with long term mental health problems. Unpublished PhD thesis, University of Nottingham, Nottingham

Quotes

This is where you refer to an author's work. You can have direct and indirect quotes.

When using direct quotes, you should also include the relevant page number(s). This allows the reader to find the original source.

BOX 10.10	*Example of direct quote*
	Pressure groups attempt to influence policy making at both national and local levels (Masterson 1994, p. 42).

BOX 10.11	*Example of an indirect quote*
	Masterson (1994) stated that one of the aims of pressure groups was to affect policy-making decisions at both local and national levels.

In both these examples, the authors would be listed in alphabetical order in the reference list.

Secondary references

Wherever possible, you should always attempt to use readily available or recent primary sources, i.e. the original publication. However, this is not always possible and you may also want to refer to a classic piece of writing that has been quoted by another author. In this case you use the term 'cited by' (a secondary reference) and the name of the author and the date of the text actually accessed.

BOX 10.12

> The role of pressure groups was outlined by Masterson (1994, cited by Maslin-Prothero 1996).
> For a secondary reference only the details of the publication accessed (i.e. Maslin-Prothero 1996) should appear in the reference list.

The Vancouver system of referencing

The Vancouver system of referencing is widely used in journals and some books. All references are identified in the text by numbers, either in brackets or as superscript. The philosophy behind this system of referencing is that the use of numbers in the text does not distract the reader by interrupting the text.

Reference to the same author and publication uses the same number. The references are then listed in numerical order.

BOX 10.13

> The World Health Organization European Region's *Targets for Health for All 2000* [1] and the British government's White Paper *The Health of the Nation* [2] both list a series of targets by which improvements in health over a specific period of time may be measured.
>
> **References**
> 1. World Health Organization (1985) *Targets for Health for All 2000.* Copenhagen: WHO Regional Office for Europe.
> 2. Department of Health (1992) *The Health of the Nation.* London, HMSO.

The style of reference for material from a book or journal is the same for Vancouver and Harvard referencing; the difference is the use of numbers in the Vancouver system.

There are a number of different referencing systems available. Each individual and institution has their preferred system of referencing. It is important that you identify the method preferred prior to submitting work, and use this method when compiling. You should check your reference to make sure it is accurate, so that should you or anyone else want to find the original source, they can.

If you are undertaking a piece of work that requires a lot of references you could choose to keep track of your references using a database, e.g. Reference Manager or EndNote, which is specifically designed for this purpose.

WRITING FOR PUBLICATION

Writing for publication provides an opportunity to share your ideas with a wider audience and is crucial if nursing is to develop and improve patient care. For those working in academic institutions, it is a fundamental requirement. If you examine the nursing press you will find that only a small number of the total nursing workforce are submitting work for publication. Masterson (1994) identified that the majority of publications and awards go to either nurses in management or nurse educators. If there is to be a more representative, balanced view of nursing then you need to contribute your thoughts and ideas to the nursing press. Learning to write is straightforward as long as you prepare and follow some simple guidelines.

Learning to write
- Identify your audience (and journal)
- Write about what you know
- Do background reading and preparation
- Use the guidelines for contributors and follow the 'house style'

From personal experience, it is worthwhile approaching the intended journal editor or publisher with your idea. Read a variety of journals and decide whether what you want to write about is suitable for that particular journal. There might be a journal that is more appropriate. For example, an article on the experience of part-time, mature midwifery/nursing students would be more suitable in *Nurse Education Today* than in the *Journal of Clinical Nursing*. Then, prepare a detailed plan of what you intend to cover and write to the editor. This will save you time because the editor can express an interest (or otherwise) in your intended published work.

Having identified the journal, use their most recent contributor guidelines when preparing the script. This will help create a favourable impression with the editor and reviewers when submitting the completed script. The guidelines for contributors include the following details: number of words, presentation issues (word processed, double-line spacing, width of margins, style of referencing), number of copies to be submitted, including floppy disc, copyright and payment. There are a number of stages you need to follow:

- the desire to write
- decide on a subject
- define your subject
- know your target journal
- approach the editor

FIGURE 10.3   *The process from submission to publication* (adapted with permission from Cook 2000)

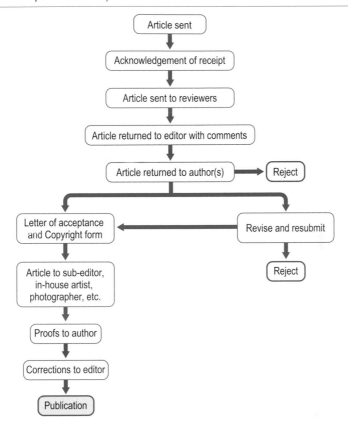

- plan the article
- write the article
- prepare for publication (Cook 2000).

Proof read your work prior to submitting it, or ask someone else to.

The editor will have your article reviewed and decide whether your manuscript is appropriate for their publication. Reviewers will comment and advise on the standard and quality of your manuscript. The reviewer will recommend one of the following: accept, some revision required, or reject. The journal editor will write to you and let you know if your work has been accepted for publication. If they recommend making some changes, and you are willing to do these, then make the changes and return the article. Once your article has been accepted the process to publication is summarized in Figure 10.3.

Be prepared for a wait of up to a year before seeing your work in print. Don't get despondent if your article is not accepted for publication. I have had work rejected, but have persevered.

CONCLUSION

This chapter has looked at presentation of written material. The main aim has been to provide you with a framework that you can use when preparing written material. This can be used in conjunction with information from other chapters for presentation of assignments, etc. It is useful to gain feedback on any written or verbal presentations you give, this will enable you to develop your skills further. You will gain in confidence and learn each time you have to submit written work.

Identify an assignment for which you have received positive feedback from your assessor. Using guidelines from a nursing journal, make necessary changes and submit it for publication.

CHAPTER RESOURCES

REFERENCES

Cook R 2000 The writer's manual: a step-by-step guide for nurses and other health professionals. Radcliffe Medical Press, Oxford

Johnson M 1995 Writing a book review: towards a more critical approach. Nurse Education Today 15: 228–231

Masterson A H R 1994 Explaining the values of British nursing and the values enshrined in United Kingdom health policy: a research proposal. Unpublished Master of Nursing Thesis, University of Wales College of Medicine, Cardiff

Watson R 1998 A message from the book reviews editor. Journal of Advanced Nursing 27: 1103

Watson R 1999 Another message from the book review editor. Journal of Advanced Nursing 29: 1283–1284

Further reading

Doyle M 1995 The A–Z of non-sexist language. Women's Press, London. *This book is an interesting and useful read. It includes a complete listing of sexist terms and their non-sexist alternatives.*

3 LEARNING FROM PRACTICE

11 Reflective skills

Elizabeth A Girot

KEY ISSUES

- **The meaning of reflection:**
  - *Personally*
  - *Professionally*
- **The process of reflection**
- **Reflection as an aid to study**
  - *Studying theory*
  - *Learning practice*
- **Types of reflection**

- **Where to start:**
  - *Critical incident analysis*
  - *Learning diaries/journals and portfolios*
  - *Developing a learning culture within the workplace*
- **The need for reflection as essential to the development of care**

INTRODUCTION

In an attempt to serve and protect the public, the Nursing and Midwifery Council (NMC) has an obligation to set and improve standards of nursing and midwifery care (Nursing and Midwifery Council 2002a). In 2002, the NMC revised the former United Kingdom Central Council for Nursing, Midwifery and Health Visiting (UKCC 2001) guidance and standards for postregistration education and practice (PREP) in the PREP Handbook (Nursing and Midwifery Council 2002b), which you may download from the NMC website (www.nmc-uk.org). One of the requirements for the achievement of these standards is for every practising nurse and midwife to compile and maintain a personal professional profile. (Guidance on how to develop your own profile can be obtained from Chapter 12.) Crucial to this is the evidence of linking your practice to study through reflection. This has been further reinforced by a number of recent Department of Health documents (e.g. 1999, 2000). In particular, the former UKCC Commission for Nursing and Midwifery Education (UKCC 1999a) reported the need to extend the use of a portfolio of practice experience to preregistration programmes to demonstrate fitness for practice, and this is reinforced in the NMC's (2002a) guidance to develop lifelong learning. Here, the use of reflection can play a vital role in preparing practitioners for professional life after registration. However, in spite of the ever-increasing body of evidence to suggest that reflective skills are crucial in making the links between theory and practice (Jarvis 1992, Murphy and Atkins 1994, Scanlan et al 2002), reflection is not as universal an activity as we think (Conway 1996, Usher et al 1999, Glaze 2002).

This chapter sets out to explore what is meant by the term 'reflection' and the skill involved in undertaking it, particularly from your personal life experiences. It will also examine ways in which you can develop the skills of reflection further to help you in the study process and to gain more from the experiences you are exposed to, both personally and professionally.

WHAT IS REFLECTION?

Jot down what you understand by the term 'reflection'.

According to Dewey (1933), people make decisions and act as a result of two types of action:

■ routine action
■ reflective action.

Routine action occurs when you 'take for granted' everyday realities of life. This 'taking for granted' allows you to concentrate on developing other aspects of your life in order to make you a more effective and efficient decision-maker. It is easy to move on to 'automatic pilot' in terms of what you do and how you do it.

Think about what you did between waking up this morning and arriving at work/university

Do you ever think about what you do in your routine activities?

Perhaps it is as well that we have such a facility as routine action; if you had to think about what you do and rethink all your decisions every day, you would be worn out! You would certainly have no energy left to make the important decisions or make decisions when faced with the unexpected. If you have learned the 'best' way of doing something, e.g. organizing yourself in the morning, driving the car, etc., then having the capacity to use this learning in an automatic way is an important facility you need to make use of.

Reflective action is concerned with weighing up all the aspects of the situation and making a conscious and informed decision about what to do. It means taking active control over what you do and how you do it. Some aspects of your everyday life depend on your use of this reflective action. However, if something works out well for you on a few occasions, it may become a routine action. If changes then occur, you may need to reconsider your automatic decisions. On the surface, this may seem a fairly straightforward concept; however, there is an increasing body of evidence to suggest that it is not quite as straightforward as we would like it to be (Moon 1999, Burns and Bulman 2000, Taylor 2003).

Moon (1999) refers to different meanings of the word reflection. She acknowledges the 'common-sense' meaning of reflection, where there can be an overlap between the use of the words 'reflection' and 'thinking'. She cites the phrases 'let me think about this one' and 'let me ponder or reflect on this' as examples of this overlap, where both phrases seem to have the same meaning. Additionally, she refers to the more academic meaning of reflection, where thinking is more critical, and describes a mental process with purpose and outcome. She suggests that the differences do not lie in the process but in the way it is used. This difference will be considered in more detail when we explore the term 'reflection' in a professional sense.

You need to use both reflective action and routine action selectively. When much of your action is routine, then you can afford to spend time evaluating other aspects of your decision making through reflective action and, once you are satisfied with your choices, these can then become 'automatic actions' for the future. However, like most situations in life, although there may be time available to evaluate the choices you make, it is often not until something unexpected happens, which prompts a sense of unease, that we are triggered to think more critically about the situation (Schon 1987, Williams 2001). Unfortunately, as Brookfield (1987) observes, most theorists emphasize the impact of negative triggers (rather than positive triggers) in prompting our need to examine issues critically.

This clearly has important implications for developing your study skills and also for developing your expertise in professional practice, which we will examine later.

Think of something significant that happened to you recently in your everyday life and that did not work out as well as you had hoped. Jot down what happened and why you think it happened the way it did. Note down how you can use this information to help you retain the knowledge and skills you are trying to learn.

It is often said that we learn from the mistakes we make. Life can be seen as a series of hurdles: each time we meet new experiences, we try to fit them into our already existing understanding to make sense of them. However, we do not always learn from our experiences. Some people are particularly self-aware and sensitive to their own response in certain circumstances, while others never seem to learn from their experiences and continue to make the same mistakes over and over again. Alternatively, you can learn to forget the experience – the experience can be too painful to explore or your feelings can be too strong to dissect. So, when you meet a similar situation in the future, it is easy to make the same mistakes over again. The learning has been one of forgetting.

There are two important issues here. First, feelings are an extremely important aspect of the learning process and the way you feel can dictate whether you learn from a particular experience or not. Feelings of anxiety or uncomfortable feelings can be a barrier to learning. Second, it is crucial that you do not learn to forget too many experiences. If this happens, making mistakes repeatedly may be extremely problematic for you, especially when there may be the opportunity of making life easier for yourself by responding in a different way.

If you find yourself repeating mistakes, perhaps you are using 'reflection' more in the way Moon (1999) refers to as the 'common-sense' meaning. That is, you are simply thinking about what you are doing and, for whatever reason, you cannot move beyond this. This is further illustrated by Box 11.1.

BOX 11.1	Often when you 'reflect' you acknowledge that something happened. You describe it to yourself, perhaps over and over again. Perhaps then you share it with someone else and this helps you see it in a different light. However, your 'reflections' often stop there. You do not allow yourself the opportunity of making sense of the situation for another time. Rather, you seem to recall it numerous times to 'get it off your chest'. Merely thinking about what you did is not in itself true reflection, certainly not at a level that requires you to make sense of it and change what you do the next time.

You have already explored some aspects of what is meant by reflection and how you can relate it to your everyday life. Although it could be argued that you are reflecting to some degree all the time, in relation to both your study skills and your professional practice, reflection as an activity is more than just thinking about what you are doing. It is about making sense of different situations and helping you to make the best choices and to incorporate them into your everyday, automatic action. In professional practice, reflection has been formalized and perhaps it would help to explore the notion of reflection in greater depth, so that you can see how to get the best out of your reflections for your professional practice.

REFLECTION IN A PROFESSIONAL SENSE

'Reflection' in professional terms takes on a particular meaning. This relates to both your study skills development and to your professional practice. In this professional sense, as Greenwood (1998) reports, there are numerous definitions of reflection (Schon 1991, Boud 1992, Mezirow 1998). Although Mackintosh (1998) acknowledges a lack of clear definition, reflection for professional practice acknowledges a way of problem solving from everyday practice. Scanlan and Chernomas (1997) argue that reflection encourages students to think critically. From a process of exploration, often triggered by a sense of the unexpected, reflection encourages you to make sense of an experience and learn from it to help you in the future. As already mentioned, feelings are a crucial element in terms of how they influence your learning from the experience.

The most important aspect of reflection is learning from the experience.

Certainly, in the current climate of enormous change in health care, both qualified practitioners and those working towards registration need to be prepared to deal with uncertainties and to find new solutions to dilemmas for each individual you care for. If individualized care is to be an accepted way of thinking about care, the lists of textbook problems in clinical practice and, even more, the recipe-book solutions to these problems, will become things of the past. Also, as an adult learner you will bring with you to the study experience your own individual ways of learning. Both for patient care and for study, you need to tailor solutions to meet individual need. It follows, therefore, that you need to find ways of helping this process to guide the activity (Moon 1999).

Before we consider different guides or 'frameworks' to help you look critically at your study or practice, it is worthwhile considering why reflection might be important for you in professional terms. Whether you are commencing or continuing your higher education study, it is hoped that through a process of lifelong learning (Nursing and Midwifery Council 2002a) from your study and your experience you will be working towards becoming an expert practitioner.

If you look around you, you can certainly identify a number of practitioners who would fit the title of expert. But what exactly do we mean by the term 'expert'? Those 'expert' practitioners whom you have identified will have a number of different attributes, yet you have identified them all as 'experts'. Conway (1996) suggests that expertise is not definitive and in her own study she identified four different types of 'expert'. She acknowledged that each type developed from their different 'world views'. These 'world views' were developed from the orientation of the expert to a number of issues, including:

- the resources available to them
- the amount of authority they were able to exercise
- their own goals and those of their organization
- the level and type of education (both professional and academic) that they had achieved
- their relationship with significant others, e.g. doctors and managers.

BOX 11.2	**Four distinct types of 'expert' identified by Conway** *(with permission from Conway 1996)*

- **Technologist:** Characterized by wide range of knowledge, including anticipatory knowledge, diagnosis knowledge, 'know-how' knowledge and monitoring knowledge both of junior doctors and patients' conditions. Teaching by these experts was mainly didactic: images were used, as was in-depth questioning and a translator function was demonstrated. Issues arose in relation to the authority that expert nurses had vis-à-vis doctors.

- **Traditionalist:** Characterized by the need for 'survival'. These experts were preoccupied with 'getting the work done' and managing care with scarce resources. For them, care had a medical focus and the experts operated as overseers and doctors' assistants. Management and doctors were perceived as all powerful. They did not value their own practice and saw themselves as powerless in terms of influence. They saw education as an optional extra and not as central to practice development. Value was attached to 'doing' and not to 'reflecting'. They showed that 'papering-over-the-cracks' was what nursing was about and this others also learned to do. This dispossessed others.

- **Specialist:** Characterized by prescribing treatment regimes, recommending medication and extending their roles. There were subdivisions within this group that reflected the traditionalists, technologists and humanistic existentialists. They had developed knowledge in terms of assessment, diagnosing, quality of life and transformative ability. Doctor–nurse relationships varied.

- **Humanistic existentialist:** Characterized by a dynamic and strong nursing focus to care. Patients were truly viewed holistically and a humanistic philosophy was used in practice. They were passionate about nursing practice. A devolved hierarchy using primary nursing was operational. Humanistic existentialist experts were risk takers. They had supportive managers, good resources and were educationally well developed. They exerted considerable power and influence and saw themselves as creating the culture in their areas. Self-awareness and reflective abilities typified this group. They were also very aware of the influence that they had on other nurses.

Interestingly, each group believed they were reflective although, in reality, this was not the case. Reflective ability was the hallmark of only one of the four types (the humanistic existentialists), with far less development in the other three groups. Their ways of thinking were different and the way they approached their practice was different, with those with minimal reflective abilities giving care that was limited in focus and illness-orientated. In contrast, reflective practitioners gave responsive care, full of warmth and based on the needs of the individual. The different 'world views' are therefore important, as they influence the 'natural' skills individuals bring to situations, with some having more advanced critical reflective skills than others.

Clearly, as Conway (1996) acknowledges, reflection in a professional sense for some, is not easy. Indeed, Moon (1999) observed from the work of student nurses Holm and Stephenson (1994) how learning to reflect was a difficult process and involved the use of skills that by no means all of the students possessed at the beginning of their programme of study. However, 5 years on, Burns and Bulman (2000) acknowledged that, through support and guidance, there was a more positive recognition by student nurses of the value of reflection and their development as curious and challenging practitioners.

In contrast to the 'thoughtful' activity described at the beginning of this chapter, reflection that encourages a change of behaviour needs to be developed and supported through a guided experience, and further supported for lifelong learning in practice.

With nursing and midwifery education firmly embedded into the world of higher education in the UK, and the development of critical thinking being the goal, Brookfield (1987) and Burton (2000) recognize the close link between the process of critical thinking development and that of reflection. This will be followed up more fully in Chapter 13.

Reflection consists of:

■ thinking about an experience
■ exploring that experience in terms of feelings and significant features
■ processing the significant features and identifying learning
■ effects of future practice.

THE PROCESS OF REFLECTION

A number of writers acknowledge the difficulties of learning from experience (Richardson and Maltby 1995, Mackintosh 1998, Scanlan et al 2002). Trying to put into words the way you processed the experience and finally learned from it is a complex activity. Helping you to think critically about your practice can be facilitated using different approaches, rather in the way that Conway (1996) described various types of expert. If you consider Conway's experts as existing along a continuum of reflective ability – from scant ability to reflect, to wholly reflective – you can identify different approaches to learning to help you, depending at which point of the reflective continuum you lie. These activities consist of frameworks such as problem-based learning (Leifer 2001, Thomas 2001, Williams 2001, Conway et al 2002, Foley 2002, McNiven et al 2002), where carefully constructed problems and questions help you to find possible solutions, and reflective cycles, where students are expected to ask their own questions and seek out problems for resolution and where analysis of their feelings is all important.

Clearly you, like those experts in Conway's study, need to find which 'world view' you subscribe to and therefore which approach will most easily help you to develop the skills of problem solving. It is hoped that, as you move through the higher education process, you will be able to not only problem solve, but to anticipate and seek out potential problems so that you can become independent in your quest for the development of critical thinking and reflection, moving towards empowerment and emancipation – at least in thought and understanding (Morrison 1995)!

As far as reflection is concerned, more and more is being written in the nursing and midwifery press about the need for reflection and offering different ways of how you might go about it in practice. Rolfe et al (2001) offer a guide to a range of available frameworks developed by different theorists, to guide you through the process (e.g. Boud et al 1985, Gibbs 1988, Johns 1998). Some are fairly detailed, others simplistic. Whatever the approach, the important factors are that you analyse your experience and learn from it. I have briefly offered a few of these frameworks for you to consider.

Structured reflection

One of the most popular frameworks to help you gain the most from your reflective action is the model of structured reflection described by Johns (1998). This framework offers a series of questions, or reflective cues, to help you to begin to understand your practice in relation to the fundamental ways of knowing identified by Carper

(1978). Johns' framework is continually being developed and is now in its 12th edition (2000) since its inception in 1992. As with any tool, it can be used to help you either think or write reflectively. The written approach is considered in Box 11.3.

BOX 11.3	*Model of structured reflection* (with permission from Johns 2000)

Looking in

- Find a space to focus on self
- Pay attention to your thoughts and emotions
- Write down those thoughts and emotions that seem significant in realising desirable work

Looking out

- Write a description of the situation surrounding your thoughts and feelings
- What issues seem significant?
- Aesthetics
  - What was I trying to achieve?
  - Why did I respond as I did?
  - What were the consequences of that for the patient/others/myself?
  - How were others feeling?
  - How did I know this?
- Personal
  - Why did I feel the way I did within this situation?
- Ethics
  - Did I act for the best? (ethical mapping)
- What factors (either embodied within me or embedded within the environment) were influencing me?
- Empirics
  - What knowledge did or could have informed me?
- Reflexivity
  - Does this situation connect with previous experiences?
  - How could I handle this situation better?
  - What would be the consequences of alternative actions for the patient/others/myself?
  - How do I now feel about this experience?
  - Can I support myself and others better as a consequence?
  - How 'available' am I to work with patients/families and staff to help them meet their needs?

Johns begins by asking you to find a space and focus on your thoughts and feelings in relation to a particular situation before writing a description of that experience. To reflect purposefully, it is important that you focus on particular aspects of the situation to prevent the purely thoughtful response described earlier in the chapter. The storytelling aspect of reflection is there as a trigger to help you tease out the issues that are important to you and with a view to learning and perhaps changing your practice, but it is only a small part of the whole process.

In Box 11.3, Johns has used Carper's four ways of knowing (Carper 1978) to help you explore different types of knowledge that inform what you do.

These ways of knowing are:

- **Empirical knowledge**: theoretical, scientific, accessible through the senses
- **Aesthetic knowledge**: artistic and creative aspects of the situation – what is most pleasing? Knowing what to do with the moment, instantly without conscious deliberation. Producing creative and deeply moving interactions with others
- **Personal knowledge**: your personal experience, which influences the situation and also how you can manage your own concerns so they do not interfere with seeing the patients
- **Ethical knowledge**: doing the 'right' thing, doing what 'ought' to be done (Chinn and Kramer 1995, pp. 4–11).

In addition to Carper's four ways of knowing, Johns constructed a fifth way of knowing, which he named 'reflexivity' and which helps you make 'sense of the present in terms of the past, with a view towards the future' (Johns 1998, p. 7). Johns suggests that there is a need for reflection to be guided, so the cues help you to stay as true to the meaning of the situation as you can. In this way, Johns encourages you to move away from the purely theoretical knowledge that you bring to each situation and explore other types of knowledge that help you make sense of the situation. This, of course, can be as relevant to your clinical practice as it is to your study. All aspects of knowing are important and contribute to the whole of knowing. Learning to articulate each aspect allows you to communicate and develop that knowledge to refine your understanding for practice.

It may be helpful to consider Johns' (2000) framework to guide your thoughts through a particular problem in your study, for example:

Imagine you set aside a particular day to work on one of your assignments for your programme of study – a whole day to write up your thoughts around all the reading you have been doing over the past few weeks. At the end of the day you feel exhausted and have very little actual writing to show for it.

So, why did you not achieve your goals? Let us just examine the issues in relation to Johns's structured reflection:

Aesthetics

What exactly were you trying to achieve? How did you plan the day? Did you break the day up into manageable sections and plan smaller goals within the day? Or did you simply start and work through the day as a whole and hope that you would complete your goals by the end? How did you keep yourself going in terms of keeping your attention and concentration?

Perhaps you set yourself unrealistic goals and the task was just too big to complete in one day? It is easy to leave assignment writing until the last moment and then find that you have left yourself too short a time to complete the work by the set deadline. One day in study terms might seem a long time, but to concentrate for the whole day is perhaps being unrealistic in terms of what you can actually achieve. This book is designed to help you begin to understand about how you learn best and how to get the most out of your reading.

As you can see from the aesthetics aspect of knowing, Johns' (2000) framework poses a number of questions, which you might like to consider, about the way you respond to the task of study and the consequences of your approach to the day.

Personal

Why did you feel the way you did about the day? Did you set out on a positive note and maintain your optimism throughout the day? Or did you feel exhausted at the thought of the task ahead and take some time to get yourself in gear for the day's activities? What influenced you in your approach to the day? Did you consider the weather and its influence on achieving your task? Did you consider the environment around you? Was it too hot or too cold? Did you plan short breaks throughout the day? Did you have enough to eat and drink (or did you spend your time making the snacks to distract you?). Were you comfortable in your seating and writing arrangements? Or were you cramped and felt muddled by the surroundings? Were there other distractions like noise, music, etc. that took your mind off what you were trying to achieve? Were you tired and anxious about the day ahead?

Ethics

Was it right that you left your complete assignment to such a late date instead of preparing yourself over a period of time? Had you completed sufficient reading to inform your writing?

Empirics

What knowledge did or could have informed you? What do you know about the theories that support the best way to learn?

Additionally, Chapter 2 in this book helps you consider how to get the best out of your efforts, about the optimum time to maintain your attention and the optimum environment to get the best out of yourself. In fact, many textbooks present the different psychological conditions that promote best learning.

Reflexivity

How does this connect with your previous experiences? How could you better handle the situation for future assignments? How could you better plan yourself to get the best out of your preparation, to achieve well in your assignments?

Applying the various thoughts that you have considered above to your own personal study habits should help you organize yourself for future events and not leave yourself vulnerable to poor-quality work just because time has run out. Also, you need to consider how you can make the most of the time that you have set aside so that the time you have is quality time, producing good-quality assignments.

So, using a guided approach, getting in touch with your feelings and responses to problems, you can learn to reflect critically and gain from your experiences. As Conway (1996) illustrated, some individuals find this easier than others. If it is not within your 'makeup' or doesn't suit your own philosophical perspective then, like any new skill, it needs practice and development, guidance and support. As students, learning the process, Holm and Stephenson (1994) present their own difficulties through their own development from a purely descriptive, storytelling approach to critical reflection. They moved on to 'find clarity and conclusion in the midst of confusion and conflict' (Holm and Stephenson 1994, p. 62). As previously mentioned, students from the same institution 5 years later offered a list of practical tips to help others struggling with the process that you might like to consider (Burns and Bulman 2000, p. 135).

The questioning approach

In an alternative approach to Johns' (2000) structured reflection, Boud et al (1985) present a more simplistic framework. This has been further modified by Driscoll (1994) to make it easier to remember in practice. Essentially, it requires you to ask yourself three questions about your particular experience:

BOX 11.4	
	■ **What?** Returning to the situation and describing it – what were the key aspects?
	■ **So what?** Understanding the context – feelings and effects of the different actions
	■ **Now what?** Modifying future outcomes – what would you change?

Each of these three questions can be subdivided into further questions, as shown in Figure 11.1 (Driscoll 1994). Although Driscoll offers you a number of reflective cues under each main question, like Johns (2000), once you have internalized the cues for yourself you can use the detailed cues to help you address the overall framework.

FIGURE 11.1

1 A *description* of the event

WHAT? trigger questions:

- is the purpose of returning to this situation?
- happened?
- did I see/do?
- was my reaction to it?
- did other people do who were involved in this?

2 An *analysis* of the event

SO WHAT? trigger questions:

- How did I feel at the time of the event?
- Were those feelings I had any different from those of other people who were also involved at the time?
- Are my feelings now, after the event, any different from what I experienced at the time?
- Do I still feel troubled, if so, in what way?
- What were the effects of what I did (or did not do)?
- What positive aspects now emerge for me from the event that happened in practice?
- What have I noticed about my behaviour in practice by taking a more measured look at it?
- What observations does any person helping me to reflect on my practice make of the way I acted at the time?

3 Proposed *actions* following the event

NOW WHAT? trigger questions:

- What are the implications for me and others in clinical practice based on what I have described and analysed?
- What difference does it make if I choose to do nothing?
- Where can I get more information to face a similar situation again?
- How can I modify my practice if a similar situation was to happen again?
- What help do I need to help me 'action' the results of my reflections?
- Which aspect should be tackled first?
- How will I notice that I am any different in clinical practice?
- What is the main learning that I take from reflecting on my practice in this way?

More recently, Kim (1999) has developed a similar method of critical reflective inquiry for nurses to develop knowledge for nursing and to improve practice. The three phases she refers to are: the Descriptive Phase (examination of what happened) – 'What?'[*my interpretation*], the Reflective Phase (analysis of the situation against existing theory) – 'So what?'[*my interpretation*] and lastly the Critical/Emancipatory Phase (demonstrating learning and a change in practice) – 'Now what?' (*my interpretation*). Here she aims to develop individual practice, nursing knowledge about practice and shared learning (Kim 1999).

Think about something in everyday life that did not work out as well as you had hoped. Use Driscoll's questions to help you analyse the situation and learn from it. Does this framework help you to alter your decision making in the future?

BOX 11.5	*Example*

A worked example of this might be your meeting with six friends to complete a joint study (agreed at a previous meeting) required for your course, and finding that you failed to achieve what you set out to do.

What? (returning to the situation)

The second meeting was arranged to complete some work as a group, which you were required to present at your next study day. You personally had completed some reading and written notes but were not quite clear as to what was expected from your contribution. At the meeting there was a great deal of argument among you, as some had completed work and others had done nothing. You were angry as you felt no one really appreciated what you had done. The key issues as you see the situation are that:

- an amount of work had been completed by three members of the group only
- the other three had done nothing
- no one was quite clear as to what had been actually agreed at the first meeting, and most had a different interpretation of what was decided at that meeting.

So what? (understanding the context)

Personal reflection: I felt angry at the time of the second meeting, as my own contribution did not seem to be valued by the others in the group. I also felt angry and resentful at the others who had not completed any work. I felt I had wasted my time.

After questioning, the three members of the group who had not completed any work were quite adamant that at the first meeting it had been decided that everyone should read around the subject matter in order to formulate a plan of action at this second meeting.

Once everyone had had the opportunity of expressing how they were feeling, it was decided to elect a group leader for this particular work so that some clear decisions could be made and documented and everyone's contribution could be clearly identified.

Learning: I now feel that we should have made this move at our first meeting. However, I am glad that we felt comfortable enough with each other to express ourselves, and it seemed to clear the air. I can now see that some of us felt quite differently from others in the group simply because of the vague discussions and decisions that were made at the first meeting. I don't feel it so surprising now that we got ourselves in such a muddle. The need to elect a leader and identify a clearly documented action plan for future work was a lesson well learned.

Now what? (modifying future outcomes)

I now see that when we are faced with a similar activity in the future, a spokesperson should be identified and each decision that is made at the meeting should be clearly documented, so that everyone knows and understands what is expected of them. I now realize that if we ignore this learning experience, we are very likely to land in a similar disorganized situation again and not be fortunate enough to have the time we had available this time to achieve our expectations. In addition, I realize that the rapport that is required to work closely together is jeopardized and the final presentation is not so likely to be successful. This is really important as I know that we will have many similar exercises to complete for other subjects. Also, I know that if everyone knows what their contribution should be for the group presentation, I personally will feel much more motivated to complete my side of the bargain.

So far, you have been concerned with decisions that have not gone according to plan. However, reflection is not just about making sense of situations when they go wrong. It is important to examine why some decisions you make are successful. You need to make sure that good decisions are repeated, rather than just changing decisions that have gone wrong.

Think of a situation in your everyday life that you felt you handled particularly well. This may be the way you handled a particularly sensitive situation with a friend who sought your advice, or it may be how you mastered a skill you have recently been working on. Why do you think you handled the situation so well? What did you say/do? What other aspects were involved that made it a success?

Again, you may like to use Driscoll's (1994) questions to help you analyse your situation in some depth. The questions should help you probe different aspects of the situation, perhaps aspects that have not readily come to mind and that at the time you felt were not significant.

This brings us on to applying what you have done so far – reflection as an everyday activity – to your study development and to learning from your professional practice. The three key stages in the whole reflective process can be summarized as follows:

BOX 11.6

1. Reflection seems to be triggered by the element of surprise (when situations turn out better than you had hoped) or by an uncomfortable feeling or thought

2. Critical analysis of the situation, involving feelings and understanding – mentally standing 'outside' yourself and using cues for guidance, ask yourself some questions about what and why you felt so uncomfortable

3. Development of a new perspective on the situation – what have you learned from this situation that would help you in the future?

REFLECTION AS AN AID TO STUDY

Studying theory

As we have already discussed, merely thinking about what you do is not in itself true reflection, certainly not at a level that will help you learn from it. It is all too easy to switch yourself on to 'automatic pilot' as far as studying is concerned and not think consciously about how you study and how you can get the best out of the time you spend studying. As you have explored using Johns' (2000) structured reflection, devoting a day of your time in pure study may give the impression of deep engagement with the theory you have in front of you. However, sitting over your books for long stretches of time may encourage you to think of other things, e.g. what might be on the television that evening, what you need to buy at the shops or how you anticipate spending your next weekend off. Routine action where study is concerned can often be time wasted. Time is precious and you need to make the most of the time you allocate to studying.

 Think of the last time you sat down to study. How much time did you spend overall? What time of the day was it and did that affect your ability to learn? How much did you feel you achieved? How could you have made better use of your time?

We all learn differently and in different ways: what might be suitable for one person is not always suitable for another. Before embarking on a programme of study, you need to identify and clarify for yourself the best way for you to learn. Ideas that might help you are developed more fully in Chapters 1 and 2. There is no right or wrong way to learn overall but, after analysing your own past experience of study, it may become clear to you what opportunities you gain from most. This is extremely important, particularly when you have to study at the same time as undertaking shift work. Knowing when, where and how you study best will help you make the most of your time.

To get the most out of your study time and the activities of reading and notetaking, you need to read Chapter 5. This will help you examine how your own pattern of study, reading and notetaking has helped or hindered you in the past. Reflecting and examining your own experiences by asking yourself questions (using cues for guidance) can now help you to improve your study for the future. Different frameworks will help provide you with cues until you can devise your own. This may take a great deal of practice and facilitation with others before you are able to do this effectively. So, do not give up!

Learning practice

Learning is not just about poring over books and learning from the written text. Much of nursing and midwifery is learned in practice. Theory and practice are closely linked; each supports the other and both are vital for successful patient care. Therefore, it is important to know how you can get the most out of your experiences in practice and learn from them.

Both nursing and midwifery practice are complex and uncertain. You are constantly being reminded of the need to develop holistic care, yet traditional textbooks are full of prescribed care that you should be offering patients. The complexities of nursing and midwifery are often not recognized by the very people who do it! When teaching colleagues about care activities, experienced practitioners often spend little time on the actual care aspects and much more on technical, procedural and medical treatments. Once it is mastered, it is as if professional care is self-explanatory and requires little thought. With the enormous amount that you are expected to learn in both pre- and postregistration programmes, some part of your programme occurs directly in practical experiences and you need to learn from these experiences. Much can be learned and taught about both the art and science of care and you will learn a lot from the experiences you are exposed to during your pre- and postregistration study programmes. To help you further, Chapter 14 is designed to give you some practical hints on how to get the most from this experience. So, to continue developing your care skills, in spite of the increasing pressures of work, consider the following questions:

- How can you make the most of your experiences in the different contexts you find yourself in?
- What is it that actually turns the experience you are getting into learning?
- Why is it that some learners appear to benefit more than others in the clinical setting?

A recent report recommending the future education requirements for midwives and nurses (UKCC 1999a) evaluated the results of the pre-registration preparation for nursing and midwifery, in higher education. With its focus on fitness for practice, it reinforces the need for the integration of theory and practice and the place of a portfolio of practice experience to provide evidence of rational decision making and clinical judgement throughout the study programmes. Alongside this report, further research (UKCC 1999b) identified that, at a postregistration level, evidence from practitioners of reflective practice within their personal professional portfolio was patchy, reinforcing the results of Conway's (1996) study that, although all practitioners believed they did reflect, this was not the case in reality. The NMC requirements for re-registration are made quite clear in their *PREP Handbook* (NMC 2002b) and this document also offers some examples from both midwifery and nursing to guide the documentation of your mandatory updating. The NMC audits compliance of this PREP (CPD) standard by sampling registrants' evidence of their learning activity and its relevance to their work (NMC 2002b). The message is clear: all practitioners need to develop much stronger links between theory and practice, and encourage a positive response to the above questions for all learners of professional practice.

Your responsibilities

There has been a move in recent years away from the traditional approach to education (giving you information and encouraging you to apply this information to a variety of circumstances) towards a much more problem-solving approach where you are expected to learn from what is happening around you. The process of 'learning how to learn' has become much more important than simply the acquisition of knowledge itself. Although the value of reflection has become a crucial element of this approach, as we have already acknowledged, it is not as straightforward as it would appear. As either a preregistration student or a qualified practitioner, you need to be encouraged to learn continuously from the 'real life' situations you face in daily practice. This may seem self-evident but it is very easy to feel so much part of the team of carers – part of the team that is required to 'get the work done' – that it is easy to lose sight of what you hope to gain from the experience. Rather like Conway's (1996) traditionalist expert, it is easy to be more concerned with getting the work done than with learning from the experience and modifying your practice as you are faced with new encounters.

What responsibility do you personally take to learn from the experiences you are faced with in the clinical setting? Do you expect to 'be taught' or do you 'actively seek to learn'? How can you improve on this?

Returning to the two types of action mentioned at the beginning of this chapter, it is very easy to switch to routine action when practising clinically. It is easy not to concern yourself with what happens, or whether decisions have been taken well or badly, especially if someone else takes the responsibility for the key decisions. However, every student and practitioner has a professional responsibility to learn to improve practice. In addition, nurse educationalists are determined to find new and innovative ways of delivering education programmes for practice, rather than encouraging the traditional theory/practice divide.

LEARNING FROM OUR MISTAKES

You will have met practitioners who have been in practice some years and have developed their practice, kept themselves up-to-date and become expert practitioners. However, you may also have had the misfortune to work with other practitioners who have been in practice for a number of years but have simply repeated their experience over time and have not learned from it.

With the drive towards more flexible career pathways and greater career opportunities from health-care assistant to consultant, coupled with the National Health Service modernization agenda advocating new ways of working and better vocational training opportunities for the wider workforce (Department of Health 1999, 2000), the boundaries between professional work and non-professional carers have become blurred. Over 10 years ago, Dewar (1992) found that first-level nurses could not differentiate easily between their own work and that of health-care assistants, and the boundaries are likely to be less clear now. You may be quite clear in your own mind what the differences are but, if challenged, could you put them into words? Perhaps the development of reflective skills will enable the profession, as a whole, to articulate the value of the professional carer. In turn, this may allow you to distinguish between you, the professional, and your assistant, and encourage you to articulate this difference in practice.

TYPES OF REFLECTION

As the concept of reflection has developed in relation to professional practice, a number of different types of reflection have been identified, i.e. in relation to reflecting before, during or after an event.

BOX 11.7

Reflecting before action

This is concerned with the variety of approaches available to you when offering patient care, planning care and anticipating the possible outcomes of a particular plan of action. Here you should be thinking about what you are about to do before you do it, and should link your already existing theoretical knowledge with the practice you are planning or implementing. Easier said than done. It is easy to understand that this should be the situation, but it is quite another thing to do it.

Reflection in action

This relates to thinking on your feet, working out what you are going to do as you are doing it. This is distinguished from routine action because you are consciously making decisions and adapting care to suit individual needs. It is sometimes called active reflection. The link between theory and practice here is much more complex and, as Conway (1996) has already demonstrated, although all 'expert' practitioners believed they were doing this, in reality, they were not.

Reflection on action

This aspect of reflection is what we have mainly been concerned about so far in this chapter. Here, you look back on your experiences and consider the success of particular interventions and decisions. The link between theory and practice may be made much more clearly some time after the event, once you have become less emotional about the situation and once you have the opportunity of analysing the situation either alone or with others. You can then consider the deeper meanings and different perspective of what was done. However, as we have already explored, there are a number of barriers to this actually happening in reality. Therefore, overall, as you develop your skills in reflecting for learning, all three types of reflection will be used.

In addition to the different types of reflecting, there are different levels of reflecting. These levels are of particular importance clinically, especially when you engage in a group discussion of an incident that happened in your work. They are also important when developing your skills of reflection for academia. These are considered briefly below.

 Learning from practice is very important in any programme of professional development, whether preregistration or postregistration. After all, the whole purpose of learning is to gain insight from our practice and to develop standards of care. Otherwise, learning and study become sterile activities.

WHERE TO START

What can you do in a practical way that will help you develop your reflective skills more formally? Three main areas will be considered here:

- the use of critical incident analysis
- learning diaries/journals and portfolios
- developing a learning culture within the workplace.

The use of critical incident analysis

Critical incidents are a way of examining a particular situation in your practice and identifying what you have learned from it. 'Critical' here refers to your critical examination of the situation. Critical incidents have been utilized in nursing for some years. More recently they have been developed for assessment purposes in both midwifery and nursing and in particular as a basis for problem-based learning activities. You might find Williams' paper (2001) useful to help your understanding of the role of problem-based learning in developing your critical reflection. As has already been mentioned, this can then enable you to develop your skills of problem solving and problem seeking for use in your personal professional profile. Although critical incidents have been associated with crisis situations, with mistakes that have been made or with poor decision making, they can and should be used for all situations, both positive and negative. In particular, Rich and Parker (1995) advocate the need for support during the process of reflection to attempt to diminish the vulnerability of the student and the lecturer and reduce anxiety.

To assist you in your own reflective analysis of your own encounters, approaches such as problem-based learning can help you develop your independence in learning and can be used to help you seek out different approaches to solving clinical problems. Problem-based learning offers you a different approach to learning, which encourages you to think critically in focused areas as well as encouraging you to go off at tangents that link up to other situations. It encourages you to read and to challenge (Williams 2001). The learning material is deliberately constructed with triggers to initiate discussion, to orientate you to course material and to confront your preconceived ideas. The role of the teacher is one of facilitator of your learning rather than fount of all knowledge (Alavi 1995). In this way, problem-based learning can help you develop your own analytical techniques when making sense of your practice.

The use of critical incident analysis is similar to any reflective analysis but is clearly related to practice. The format for working through the analytical process can be wide and varied. Indeed, you can devise your own way of analysing the situation. Alternatively, the frameworks that were considered earlier (Boud et al 1985, Johns 2000) may be helpful or, additionally, the following might be more helpful:

- Describe the situation
- Examine the components of the situation – the key issues/roles
- Analyse your feelings about the situation – how you felt then, how you feel now
- Analyse what you know of this aspect of practice – the alternatives available to you
- Challenge any assumptions you have made
- Explore how you might change or confirm your approach for the next time.

The nature of knowledge

It is important to recognize that knowledge gained for practice does not just come from textbooks. Burns and Bulman (2000) note that nursing and midwifery knowledge has been classified in various ways. Carper's (1978) four ways of knowing is well known in nursing and is used by Johns (2000) in his structured model of reflection. However, Clarke and Keeble (1995) identify five main sources of nursing and midwifery knowledge:

- Science
- Tradition
- Ritual
- Common sense
- Authority.

Think of a situation that occurred in your own practice recently. It may be a routine activity that you felt you handled particularly well or something that sticks in your mind as special in some way. Using the framework identified for critical incident analysis, identify any new knowledge you have gained from the experience and where you obtained this knowledge from.

The skill of integrating new knowledge with previous knowledge is important in all our development and helps us to individualize the care we give and to improve the standards of care overall. It is an important skill, enabling reflection to help us to adapt care in new situations and change our thinking about the way we do things.

Learning diaries/journals and portfolios

Increasingly, programmes of study encourage students to complete reflective diaries of learning experiences. The purpose of these is to help you understand yourself – your strengths and limitations, the opportunities that were available to you and the threats to your development. Diaries help you to describe your experiences, to analyse the different processes contributing to the decision making and, through learning, to develop your practice. A diary will help you to bring together the theory you have been reading and learning with the practice in clinical placements (see Chapter 12). A diary is about reflecting: thinking, analysing and learning are the key skills to a successful diary and portfolio. It is much more than simply telling the story. Although reflection is a skill that needs to be learned, the more you examine and explore your practice, the easier it should become to probe deeper into the complexities of your practice and begin to tease out the different issues. Knowing the 'right' questions to ask yourself is a crucial stage in this probing exercise.

As mentioned earlier, since April 1995, in spite of an obligation for all qualified practitioners to complete their own personal professional profile in order to re-register, evidence of reflective practice has been patchy (UKCC 1999b). For the purpose of monitoring linkage to practice for maintaining registration, the NMC (Nursing and Midwifery Council 2002b) has published its intention to monitor PREP compliance by registered midwives and nurses. The role of reflection is crucial to provide the evidence for this link and so it is important that you as a professional, or as someone seeking registration, are supported in some way to improve your reflective skills.

Nevertheless, a number of constraints to the effective implementation of reflection have been recognized. Among these are lack of time to complete the activity, lack of support to implement changes in practice and lack of skills of critical analysis in the documentation of this reflection (Heath 1998). In fact, Heath offers a practical guide to keeping a reflective diary, suggesting that one side of the page is given to telling the 'story' while the other side is used for reflection and analysis notes. In this way, the points raised in the descriptive diary are addressed in some way on the other side of the page, answering your self-posed question of 'So what? – what point am I trying to make in relation to confirming my good practice or suggesting change?' Heath also recommends that you should undertake reflection without sticking to a rigid framework, rather using your own imagination and creativity as to the problem identification and its solutions. Frameworks can then be used as a checklist after reflecting to add further dimensions and depth of thought. Alternatively, they can help get you started by offering a range of questions to ask yourself.

For the purpose of your learning diary or personal professional profile, the presentation of reflective accounts of your study and practice need not be lengthy tomes but short, analytical accounts of what you gained from the experience. However, it is not until you become practised in teasing out the points for analysis in your 'stories' that you can become skilled at focusing and become more adept at identifying your learning.

Finally, it is well recognized that reflection for better decision making can indeed be a painful and isolating experience:

> In the varied topography of professional practice, there is a high, hard ground where practitioners can make effective use of research-based theory and technique, and there is a swampy lowland where situations are confusing 'messes' incapable of technical solution. The difficulty is that the problems of the high ground, however great their technical interest, are often relatively unimportant to clients or to the larger society, while in the swamp are the problems of greatest human concern.
>
> (Schon 1991, p. 42)

This difficulty needs to be recognized by us all. It is the 'messy' areas that pose the greatest challenge to us and it is crucial, therefore, to gain support in both analysing the situations and identifying possible solutions. This will be considered in more detail in the next section.

Developing a learning culture/learning community within the workplace

Many writers have identified the shortcomings of reflecting on your own (Newell 1992, Jones 1996, Wallace 1996, Burns & Bulman 2000).

They recognize the problems of the effect of memory on the reflector (Wallace 1996), the uncertainties of accuracy (Newell 1992) and the problems of possible misinterpretation of events (Jones 1996). However, reflection need not be a solitary activity. In fact, it could be argued that there is only so much you can learn when reflecting on your own.

As reflection is now an integral part of each practitioner's development, and particularly given its value within the context of the government's agenda on clinical governance (Royal College of Nursing 1998, Heath and Freshwater 2000), everyone has an obligation to monitor their own performance and show evidence of learning. Reflection can be extremely time-consuming and laborious, or it can be pleasurable and profitable. It is up to you to make the most of the opportunities that present themselves and gain from your experiences. Part of that may be finding the right person to help you through your thought processes.

Driscoll (1994) refers to a learning culture within the workplace and Rolfe et al (2001) to a learning community. These simply mean that enjoying and sharing learning within your workplace becomes part of the 'norm'. Then, in turn, you might document some of the most meaningful reflections in your personal professional profile.

More emphasis seems to be being placed on the importance of sharing your reflections in practice. Formal roles have been devised and formal structures implemented to aid the process.

Think of the formal roles and structures that are in progress in your own area of practice, or that you are aware of, and identify whether they are successful or not. You might now explore why they are so successful (or not!).

Formal roles such as mentoring, preceptorship and clinical supervision are relatively recent innovations within nursing and midwifery, being introduced in the late 1970s. Peer support is another way of seeing these roles – they are most definitely not authoritarian structures. However, they are a way of formalizing support that has always been an implicit system among health care professionals. However, Heath and Freshwater (2000, p. 1298) argue the need for a well planned process with a well-prepared supervisor to permit a 'move towards independence, emancipation and evolving expertise'. Butterworth et al (1998) argue that using a variety of approaches to seeking and gaining support in the workplace, such as peer group and network supervision, make support accessible and accepted as an established part of healthcare work.

The success of the roles and structures of support is dependent on the ability and commitment of the individuals themselves, as well as on the preparation and resources available to fulfil the roles as they were designed. Shared reflections within a trusting relationship are an important ingredient to the success of these roles. Unfortunately, short placements, resource constraints and sometimes a misunderstanding of each other's roles are causes for concern and prevent their greater success.

Individual performance appraisal is another structure that allows the opportunity of reflecting on your experience over the last year with your manager and identifying your aspirations for the coming year, in line with departmental/trust policy. To get the most out of this appraisal, you need to work hard at your reflections and encourage positive discussion about how well you are progressing and how your manager can help you fulfil your aspirations.

Listening

One of the greatest qualities you can have to help someone in their reflections is the skill of listening. It is easy to interrupt a colleague or friend when they are exploring a situation that happened to them with a similar experience that you have had yourself. Resist the temptation and encourage your colleague to explore the situation deeply. You can provide the cues and the questioning skills to help them to do so. It can be satisfying and fulfilling to participate in another's reflective activities, as well as to share your own experiences. You can learn as much as they can from the situation from being a more objective observer of the situation. When several of you have been involved in the same situation, you should consider finding the opportunity of sharing the different perspectives of the situation together. It may surprise you to discover the different perspectives and lessons that have been learned by each of you.

WHY REFLECT?

We have explored the difference between routine action and reflective action and how each can help you get the most out of your experiences. It is important to clarify when it is appropriate to use each. You cannot survive without some routine action, but neither can you survive effectively without reflective action. The two combine to help you along the road to becoming an expert practitioner. Studying and learning from practice must be balanced. It is important to remember that thinking about what you are doing is a natural activity that you carry out every day. Critical reflection is much more difficult. It is more analytical and encourages a more in-depth examination of your practice. It is a skill that you need to work through with support. From Conway's (1996) work we have seen that not all experts find reflection easy; we are not all natural reflectors. However, those who can develop the skill will go on to become more informed practitioners.

Much has been written about the theory–practice gap but little headway has been made as to how this gap can be narrowed. Perhaps the recent response from the profession towards developing the reflective practitioner (where learning has its foundation in practice and theory is developed out of practice) will provide a more united approach to this elusive issue.

Burns and Bulman (2000) discuss emancipation through critical enquiry. This emancipation can be both personal, for you as an individual, as well as professional, for the professions as a whole. Perhaps through the development of shared reflections, where perspectives are recognized, the professions can begin this emancipation. It is hoped that the subsequent shared and supportive environment will enrich your practice and, in time, the professions will be better enabled to articulate its value, as well as to draw together the theory and the practice of nursing and midwifery for the development of care for clients.

CONCLUSION

This chapter links closely with the previous chapters and has been designed to help you develop your understanding of how reflection can be used to help you study and, in particular, to help you gain as much as you can from both your study and your clinical practice. By attempting to make sense of both the term and the process of reflection, the chapter aims to demonstrate how meaningful reflection can help you in both a personal and professional way. A number of types of reflection, as well as a range of reflective frameworks, are available to help you understand the meaning of how and what you do, so that you can advance your work and practice and not make the same mistakes over and over. Although reflection is not easy, the practical suggestions in this chapter, e.g. critical incident analysis and learning diaries, and the development of a learning culture/community within the workplace, will help you progress through your journey.

- You need to distinguish between automatic action and reflective action, and consider when each is appropriate in both your study and your practice.
- Reflection can be valuable both personally and professionally. You need to reflect on how you can make the most of your reflections for successful learning.

- There are different ways of reflecting. You need to find the best way for you.
- There are different types of reflection. As you become more skilled you will find yourself developing the skills of each type of reflection.
- Different ways have been identified to help you to start reflecting on your experiences.

- Discuss with your friends what they mean by reflection and how they go about it.
- Discuss with your colleagues/mentor how you could share your reflections about aspects of care that several of you are involved in. Perhaps there is a time in the day/week that you could find to undertake this.
- When something out of the ordinary happens, reflect on it and see what you have learned. Discuss it with someone else involved. Write it down.
- Read some of the references to find other 'ways'/structures to help you examine your practice more easily and learn from it.

CHAPTER RESOURCES

REFERENCES

Alavi C (ed) 1995 Problem-based learning in a health sciences curriculum. Routledge, London

Boud D 1992 In the midst of experience: developing a model to aid learners and facilitators. In: Harris R, Willis P (eds) Striking a balance. Centre for Human Resource Studies, University of South Australia, SA Branch, AAACE, pp. 267–272

Boud D, Keogh R, Walker D (eds) 1985 Reflection: turning experience into learning. Kogan Page, London

Brookfield S 1987 Developing critical thinkers. Challenging adults to explore alternative ways of thinking and acting. Open University Press, Buckingham

Burns S, Bulman C (eds) 2000 Reflective practice in nursing: the growth of the professional practitioner, 2nd edn. Blackwell Science, Oxford

Burton AJ 2000 Reflection: nursing's practice and education panacea? Journal of Advanced Nursing 31: 1009–1017

Butterworth T, Faugier J, Burnard P 1998 Clinical supervision and mentorship in nursing, 2nd edn. Stanley Thornes, Cheltenham

Carper B 1978 Fundamental patterns of knowing in nursing. Advances in Nursing Sciences 1: 13–23

Chinn P, Kramer M 1995 Theory and nursing: a systematic approach, 4th edn. Mosby, St Louis, MO

Clarke E, Keeble S 1995 Sources of nursing and midwifery knowledge. South Bank University, London

Conway J 1996 Nursing expertise and advanced practice. Quay Books, Salisbury
Conway J, Little P, McMillan M 2002 Congruence or conflict? Challenges in implementing problem-based learning across nursing cultures. International Journal of Nursing Practice 8: 235–239
Department of Health 1999 Making a difference: strengthening the nursing, midwifery and health visiting contribution to health and healthcare. The Stationery Office, London
Department of Health 2000 A health service of all the talents: developing the NHS workforce. The Stationery Office, London
Dewar B 1992 Skill muddle? Nursing Times 12(88): 24–27
Dewey D 1933 How we think. DC Health & Co, Boston, MA
Driscoll J 1994 Reflective practice for practice. Senior Nurse 13: 47–50
Foley J 2002 Problem based learning: an exploratory literature review. All Ireland Journal of Nursing and Midwifery 2: 43–47
Gibbs G 1988 Learning by doing. A guide to reading and learning methods. Further Education Unit, Oxford Polytechnic, Oxford
Glaze J 2002 Stages in coming to terms with reflection: student advanced nurse practitioners' perceptions of their reflective journeys. Journal of Advanced Nursing 37: 265–272
Greenwood J 1998 The role of reflection in single loop and double loop learning. Journal of Advanced Nursing 27: 1048–1053
Heath H 1998 Keeping a reflective practice diary: a practical guide. Nurse Education Today 18: 592–598
Heath H, Freshwater D 2000 Clinical supervision as an emancipatory process: avoiding inappropriate intent. Journal of Advanced Nursing 32: 1298–1306
Holm D, Stephenson S 1994 Reflection – a student's perspective. In: Palmer A, Burns S, Bulman C (eds) Reflective practice in nursing: the growth of the professional practitioner. Blackwell Scientific, Oxford, pp 53–62
Jarvis P 1992 Reflective practice and nursing. Nurse Education Today 12: 174–181
Johns C 1998 Opening the doors of perception. In: Johns C, Freshwater D (eds) Transforming nursing through reflective practice. Blackwell Science, Oxford, pp 1–20
Johns C 2000 Becoming a reflective practitioner: a reflective and holistic approach to clinical nursing, practice development and clinical supervision. Blackwell Science, Oxford
Jones P R 1996 Hindsight bias in reflective practice: an empirical investigation. Journal of Advanced Nursing 21: 783–788
Kim HS 1999 Critical reflective inquiry for knowledge development in nursing practice. Journal of Advanced Nursing 29: 1205–1212
Leifer D 2001 The problem is . . . . Nursing Standard 16(2): 15
Mackintosh C 1998 Reflection: a flawed strategy for the nursing profession. Nurse Education Today 18: 553–557
McNiven P, Kaufman K, McDonald H 2002 A problem-based learning approach to midwifery. British Journal of Midwifery 10: 75–75
Mezirow J 1998 On critical reflection. Adult Education Quarterly 48: 185–198
Moon J 1999 Reflection in learning and professional development. Kogan Page, London
Morrison K 1995 Dewey, Habermas and reflective practice. Curriculum 16: 82–94
Murphy K, Atkins S 1994 Reflection with a practice-led curriculum. In: Palmer A, Burns S, Bulman C (eds) Reflective practice in nursing: the growth of the professional practitioner. Blackwell Scientific, Oxford, ch 1, pp 10–19
Newell R 1992 Anxiety, accuracy and reflection: the limits of professional development. Journal of Advanced Nursing 17: 1326–1333
Nursing and Midwifery Council 2002a Supporting nurses and midwives through lifelong learning. NMC, London

Nursing and Midwifery Council 2002b The PREP handbook: protecting the public through professional standards. NMC, London

Rich A, Parker D L 1995 Reflection and critical incident analysis: ethical and moral implications of their use within nursing and midwifery education. Journal of Advanced Nursing 22: 1050–1057

Richardson G, Maltby H 1995 Reflection on practice: enhancing student learning. Journal of Advanced Nursing 22: 235–242

Rolfe G, Freshwater D, Jasper M 2001 Critical reflection for nursing and the helping professions: a user's guide. Palgrave, Hampshire

Royal College of Nursing 1998 Guidance for nurses on clinical governance. RCN, London

Scanlan J M, Chernomas W M 1997 Developing the reflective teacher. Journal of Advanced Nursing 22: 235–242

Scanlan J, Care D, Udod S 2002 Unravelling the unknowns of reflection in classroom teaching. Journal of Advanced Nursing 38: 136–143

Schon D A 1987 Educating the reflective practitioner. Basic Books, New York

Schon D A 1991 The reflective practitioner: how professionals think in action. Avebury, Aldershot

Taylor C 2003 Narrating practice: reflective accounts and the textual construction of reality. Journal of Advanced Nursing 42: 244–251

Thomas G 2001 The possibilities of problem based learning in midwifery. Practising Midwife 4: 42

UKCC 1999a Fitness for practice: the UKCC commission for nursing and midwifery education. UKCC, London

UKCC 1999b UKCC PREP monitor project: summary report. UKCC, London

UKCC 2001 The PREP handbook. UKCC, London

Usher K, Francis D, Owens J 1999 Reflective writing: a strategy to foster critical enquiry in undergraduate nursing students. Australian Journal of Advanced Nursing 17: 7–12

Wallace D 1996 Using reflective diaries to assess students. Nursing Standard 10(36): 44–47

Williams B 2001 Developing critical reflection for professional practice through problem-based learning. Journal of Advanced Nursing 34: 27–34

Useful websites

Department of Health: www.dh.gov.uk

Institute of Learning and Teaching: www.ilt.ac.uk

Nursing and Midwifery Council: www.nmc-uk.org; www.nmc-uk.org/ nmc/main/publications/lifelong.pdf

12 Developing a portfolio

Liz Redfern with Anne Palmer

KEY ISSUES

- The language of portfolios
- Portfolio learning
- Ground rules for portfolio development
- Getting started
- Maintaining portfolios
- Assessing portfolios

INTRODUCTION

This chapter offers a practical guide to portfolios – what they are, how to keep one, guidelines for assessment and, perhaps most importantly, how to learn from developing your portfolio. As you may be aware, a portfolio is more than a record of events, experiences or career developments. It is a vital, 'living' document that has a secure and respected place within mechanisms for professional regulation and continuing professional development. It encourages us to make sense of what we are doing and to learn through reflection. Developing a portfolio enables you to:

- celebrate your achievements
- target your professional development
- develop your skills of learning from experience
- make decisions for the future based on the knowledge of the past.

To assist learning, as you read through this chapter, connections will be made with other chapters in the book.

Find an image or a picture from a postcard, magazine, journal or newspaper that best reflects how you feel about keeping a portfolio.

Having found your image, examine it and consider the following, making a note of your deliberations.

- Describe the image in words
- What does the image say about your feelings concerning keeping a portfolio?
- How would you classify your feelings?
- Ask yourself why you should have these feelings
- How do you intend dealing with your feelings?

Just because portfolios are seen as an integral aspect of modern learning and professional regulation (Nursing and Midwifery Council 2001) it does not necessarily mean that everyone will feel positive about keeping one. It is important to identify and acknowledge your thoughts and feelings about such a process if you are to do it well. You may have taken a minimalist approach to this, hoping the Nursing and Midwifery Council (NMC) never ask for evidence of your portfolio when you re-register. You may be someone who has thrown their heart and soul into keeping a portfolio because you have always had a tendency to write about your everyday experiences as a way of understanding yourself and the world around you – or like most readers, you may be somewhere in between.

WHAT IS A PORTFOLIO?

A portfolio is a collection of your experiences and learning activities that demonstrates your personal and professional development. Keeping a portfolio allows you to document what you are doing and, just as importantly, what you are learning. As Gibbs (1992) suggests, this record makes it easier to explain what you are doing to others and adds credibility both to your actions and to your learning.

For practitioners busy in the world of practice and for student nurses and midwives the issue of portfolios and profiles may initially appear confusing, raising such questions as 'What are they?', 'Why do I need one?' and 'What do I put in one?'. Sensible enough questions, given the terminology and 'jargon' that tends to proliferate when new concepts about learning are introduced to the professional workplace. It is always useful to begin with the basics and to gain an understanding and appreciation of what such concepts are concerned with, and what the expectations are for both you and the profession.

The rationale

The rationale for the introduction of portfolios and profiles arose from a variety of pressures in the contemporary world of work. These included the need to assist practitioners to make sense of learning experiences in practice (experiential learning) and to make connections with planned learning (courses, in-service training, conferences or workshops). Another major influence has been the increasing trend towards work-based vocational and professional learning where it is necessary to keep portfolios of evidence about what is being learnt as part of an on-going, continuous process. However, perhaps the strongest influences have arisen from the need for a 'grown up' professional regulatory framework which trusts the individual registered practitioner to be accountable for their own updating and lifelong learning (Nursing and Midwifery Council 2001). This is all in the context of increasing professional autonomy, public accountability and new quality frameworks in the guise of clinical governance.

These influences have led to explorations and requirements to record learning and individual professional development as a meaningful process. It is generally agreed that this process should encourage further learning and facilitate professional accreditation. This accreditation is the process that offers recognition to a practitioner's experience and professional competence (Hull and Redfern 1996).

The notion of keeping a record in the form of a portfolio arises from such educational theories and approaches as experiential learning, self-directed learning, problem-based learning and the more recent development of portfolio-based learning (portfolio learning; see Chapter 2). These educational theories and approaches place the learner at the centre of an active process of learning, with individuals taking responsibility for identifying and reflecting on the diversity of learning opportunities that present. These learning opportunities include:

- exploring the everyday experiences that we have
- examining critical incidents
- making mistakes
- discussions with peers
- observing alternative ways of doing things through visits and shadowing others
- having the benefit of mentors, preceptors and clinical supervisors.

The portfolio is a document containing a collection of evidence that demonstrates your personal and professional achievements, while portfolio learning is the process of recording and working with your writing (Pietroni and Millard 1996). Portfolio learning is much more than good record keeping, it is more concerned with how you engage with your thoughts and ideas. It involves collecting the evidence, analysing your learning opportunities or working through critical incidents (see Chapter 9).

A portfolio provides a safe environment, controlled by you, where you can be free to:

- acknowledge and build on your strengths
- confront your weaknesses or fears
- add perspective and depth to what you do.

In the past, nurses have not always been forthright in marketing their skills effectively or in valuing their contribution to the healthcare team. Engaging in portfolio learning can be a useful stage in developing self-awareness and building confidence and professional insights.

Portfolio learning involves:

■ focusing on your experiences

■ collecting and organizing evidence

■ analysing critical incidents

■ having a critical dialogue with yourself (see Chapter 9)

■ working with your ideas and entries

■ acknowledging what you are learning and feeling

■ making connections with what you are learning

The language of portfolio learning has been made more confusing in nursing than perhaps it might have been had the statutory and professional bodies arrived at a consensus for the documentation of professional achievement. As it evolved and prior to the creation of the NMC, the various national boards prepared versions with the 'Professional Profile' (Welsh National Board); 'Professional Portfolio' (English National Board) and 'Personal Professional Profile' (UKCC). The Royal College of Nursing (1990) provided a 'Professional Portfolio' and the *Nursing Times* a 'Portfolio Pack' (Palmer 1993). Without an appreciation of the links between the documentation and portfolio learning, it is perhaps not surprising that many practitioners and would-be practitioners felt confused (Payne 1999).

THE LANGUAGE OF PORTFOLIOS

Brown (1995, p. 89) is clear in offering a useful glossary of terms in which a 'personal portfolio is a private collection of evidence which demonstrates learning and application to professional practice', whereas a personal profile is 'selected evidence from the portfolio which demonstrates learning for a specific purpose'.

As Hull and Redfern (1996) suggest, the manner in which the various terms are used should be derived from their particular purpose.

The portfolio, then, is the overall collection of evidence for personal and professional development, while the profile is evidence, drawn from your portfolio, that you choose to share for a specific purpose such as a job interview or making the case for gaining credit in higher education (which takes the form of Accreditation of Prior Learning – APL and Accreditation of Experiential Learning – APEL; see Chapter 13). The profile can also be used for the purpose of professional accreditation with the requirement of a record of personal and professional achievement – 'the personal professional profile'. This is a flexible, comprehensive account of your professional development and how this has been accomplished.

As was discussed earlier, it should be appreciated that a portfolio is a recognizable and tangible part of portfolio learning, which concerns the collecting, writing-up and analysing of experiences and significant learning. Portfolio development is concerned with reflecting on your experiences and making the links between personal insights, personal experiences and professional practice (see Chapters 11 and 14). It is not by chance that portfolios are increasingly being used in educational programmes, in practice, for accreditation and by a variety of other health professionals (Routledge et al 1997).

The emerging evidence suggests that, in order to survive in an increasingly technological and consumer-focused environment, professional practitioners will need to be competent, critical thinkers who continually update themselves. Employers expect professionals to be lifelong learners who will change and grow as the organization changes and grows. Indeed many employers in the public and private sector talk about their employees as 'human capital' in the same way as they might describe other assets such as buildings. The staff employed in the NHS, which still sees periods of no or low growth in the way it is funded, are its greatest asset, especially through their ability for growth through learning.

Portfolio learning and developing a portfolio can be seen as an important part of the 'educational jigsaw' that underpins the notion of the learning individual as someone committed to lifelong learning. This is demonstrated in Figure 12.1, where the learning theories, approaches and professional support systems that are integral to encouraging practitioners to become learning individuals are set alongside one another.

Each theory or approach has an important part to play in providing the overall 'picture' and in helping you to take responsibility for learning from your experiences and making the most of each learning opportunity that presents. A brief overview of the individual theories and approaches is presented in Table 12.1, which identifies the various terms in current use with their practical application (see Chapter 11).

Having located portfolios within the current repertoire of learning activities it becomes easier to appreciate the purpose of portfolios in the professional world of work. As demonstrated in Figure 12.1,

FIGURE 12.1 *The learning theories, approaches and professional support systems integral to developing the learning individual* (adapted from Palmer 2000).

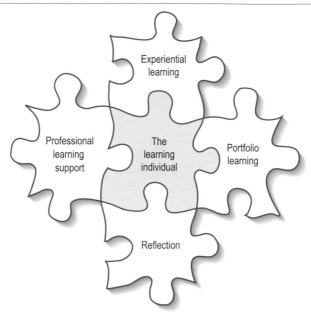

portfolios are an important feature of continuing professional education. Wilkin (undated) summarizes the key purposes as:

- Providing a record of individual professional development
- Providing recognition of achievement, strengths and commitment
- Linking individual development with organizational development
- Developing the reflective culture of an organization
- Facilitating the collection and collation of a range of information
- Providing a resource for reflection with a mentor, preceptor or clinical supervisor.

These are useful purposes that allow you to celebrate your achievements, target your professional development, develop your skills as a learning individual and gain confidence in your abilities (Palmer 2000). There need to be some ground rules for constructing a portfolio and those that are evident in good educational practice are identified in the discussions that follow.

As Dewing (1990) identifies, the portfolio is the property of the nurse who writes it. Each individual is free to reveal only what they want to, and this is important when the more reflective elements of

TABLE 12.1	An overview of educational theories and approaches relating to the learning individual

Theory/approach	Application
Experiential learning	**Creating a desire to know more**
Concerns developing your problem-solving abilities, taking responsibility for your part in the learning process and learning from experience	Involves thinking critically by challenging your assumptions and the assumptions of others. It includes identifying, planning and evaluating your learning opportunities
Reflection	**Developing abilities to integrate knowledge and find meaning within practice**
Concerns the thinking about, mulling over and working through of ideas, issues and critical incidents	Involves exploring feelings and learning from practice by examining and recording actions, leading to new insights and effective practice
Professional learning support	
Concerns the significant others who support and encourage us by being accessible, approachable and competent. These are the mentors, preceptors and clinical supervisors who help us to reflect and assist our professional development	**Working with critical friends**
	Involves the building of enabling relationships that are built on mutual trust and respect to provide a supportive environment where we can consider our practice
Portfolio learning	**Working with your ideas and entries**
Concerns the regular maintenance of a portfolio that documents and draws together your experiences and provides reflections on practice	Writing up and engaging with the entries is important. This allows for further learning and allows you to demonstrate your personal and professional achievements in an organized manner

a portfolio are considered. Johns (2000, p. 44) believes that reflecting on experience focuses attention on a meaningful event and that the writing up of these accounts in a journal or diary creates a space 'to focus on self – to look in on self and acknowledge who we are' (see Chapter 11).

Such reflections are commonly recorded in parts of a portfolio that are variously described in the literature as the reflective journal or diary, the learning journal or learning log. Others identify 'think books' or 'work books', which document materials written over time that go beyond describing and reviewing events (Moon 1999). What is common to all these descriptions is that they are an essential component of the portfolio process, as they provide an interpretive and narrative account of experience and contain sensitive, as well as confidential, material. The names are perhaps not so important as the activities that engage you with your learning and experiences in a meaningful way. What is also important is that you are offered a clear explanation of what is expected from you in writing these narratives, particularly if your portfolio is to be assessed.

It is good practice to include the reflective elements and other sensitive information in the private section of your portfolio. This remains confidential to you, although, as part of your professional development and in reflecting upon your practice, you may choose to share some aspects of this section with a trusted colleague. It is also essential that information from a portfolio should not be shared or revealed without the consent (preferably written) of the author. This becomes particularly important when portfolios become part of the assessment process, as will be discussed later.

GROUND RULES FOR SUCCESSFUL PORTFOLIO BUILDING

- Your portfolio is your personal document
- The information should be accessible and owned by you
- The content can be flexible and creative but it should be organized to make sense to you
- You should be able to provide evidence to support your deliberations
- Your learning and professional development should be related to your practice
- Your portfolio should include a self-appraisal of professional development
- Regular maintenance is essential to keep a record up to date and relevant
- The contents are confidential and you need only reveal what you wish to
- Keep your portfolio in a safe place as it may contain sensitive information about you and others

The last two points are important to allow you to engage with what you write, ask critical questions of yourself and reflect on how you are performing. The use of critical incidents can form a vital part of your portfolio development and you need to be aware that others could take incidents and events out of context. Another aspect that arises from these last two points concerns how you maintain your portfolio. It will become a living part of your practice and encourage individual learning if you consider linking some of your deliberations to staff development initiatives such as your appraisal or individual performance review.

As demonstrated in Figure 12.1 and Table 12.1, sharing some elements of your portfolio with your clinical supervisor or mentor can also assist you in making sense of your developing self-awareness and professional growth (Morton-Cooper and Palmer 2000). How you do this is entirely up to you but it is preferable if you begin to make connections between your performance, professional support and any staff development that is available to you. This is sound advice for students on educational programmes where personal tutors, module leaders or academic supervisors are on hand to assist with learning and reflecting. It is certainly worth contemplating how others can assist with the process of your portfolio learning.

Having identified what portfolios are and having considered some ground rules for developing a portfolio, the time has come to make a start.

GETTING STARTED

It is important to recognize that many nurses have trouble in making a start on developing a portfolio. In workshops around the UK practitioners and students have shared that they are too busy, that they don't see the point and wouldn't have a clue what to record or collect.

If something is preventing you making a start then you should work with the issues that emerged from the activity on page 257. This can be helpful in making you more confident about your portfolio and in taking control of the processes involved. There are many reasons why people have strong feelings about portfolios and, once again, the case studies demonstrate some of these. A sensible approach in starting is to consider the purpose for the portfolio that you are being asked to keep. This is particularly important if you are developing or maintaining one for professional development purposes and accreditation of practice.

It is a good idea to examine what is required in terms of the structure or guidelines offered to help you. There is no formula about where to start. This is a very individual to you. Wherever it makes sense to start to you is the right place to start. It may be easier to start with what you already know and any information that you have already collected about yourself. For many of us this will be factual information concerning our academic and professional qualifications, career history and the courses or study days we have attended. Others will have a curriculum vitae or course certificates and these should also be included. It is important to remember that the portfolio is much more than a factual record of employment or career progression.

You will be expected to record significant experiences and, more importantly, demonstrate the learning from those experiences. Some of the portfolios that have been developed by publishers are organized into useful sections and are especially helpful if you are not sure of how to structure a portfolio.

The NMC (Nursing and Midwifery Council 2001) describes compiling a portfolio as a continuous process, which includes three steps:

Step 1: Reviewing your experience to date
Step 2: Self-appraisal
Step 3: Setting your goals and action plans.

MAINTAINING A PORTFOLIO

Having started in this way the common concerns and issues shared among nurses mainly concern questions of 'There is too much for me to identify' and 'How do I make my records manageable?' These may become much less of an issue for some of you if you work through a prepared portfolio (the ready-made examples produced by individual Trusts and certain publishers) or read more about portfolios.

What you do need to bear in mind are the guidelines that may have been offered, both by the NMC and by any educational programme you are attending. It is always good practice to pay attention to these but you should understand and 'own' them to help you celebrate your achievements. If you are short of time or not feeling particularly creative then you should consider the range of structured portfolios that are available, which include those for the personal computer.

As noted earlier, the NMC's 'Personal Professional Profile' should contain at least two sections. The first should contain confidential information, which is personal documentation that is private and does not have to be shared. The second section should contain the information that is a requirement for professional accreditation. However, it is left to you to be creative and decide what information and evidence you need and how you want to organize the material.

In maintaining a portfolio you need to remember that this is your personal document, owned by you, and it needs to demonstrate what you are capable of. It is your own safe space where you have complete freedom to reflect on your actions. The discipline of recording your thoughts aids reflection and, as Moon (1999) identifies, writing:

- encourages you to organize and clarify your thoughts, which in turn improves understanding
- focuses your attention and actively engages you with learning
- helps you appreciate whether you know something or not

- facilitates a deeper and more active approach to learning, as you seek to explore and explain things
- slows your thought processes, allowing you to capture your thoughts and ideas for further consideration
- allows you to record your thoughts and put these in context
- encourages you to be creative and develop new frameworks.

A great deal of time can be wasted on deciding what activities to include and what not to include, with the result that the focus is on courses attended and irrelevant material. We would support Vousdon's (2000, p. 29) sensible verdict that 'the activity itself is almost irrelevant, what counts is the way in which you can show that you're a better practitioner as a result of it'.

In maintaining a portfolio you need to work with and engage with what you write, making learning an active process. It is a good idea to write regularly and to use highlighter pens, pictures, photographs, cartoons, cuttings or anything that captures what you are thinking about. As Vousdon suggests, it is working with the material you are collating and its relevance to your practice that is important, not neat rows of courses that may have limited meaning for you and assessors.

The process of working with your entries in your portfolio is illustrated in Figure 12.2.

This process should consist of a continual cycle of:

- recording and reviewing an activity
- reflecting on and identifying the learning that has been achieved
- demonstrating the implications of this learning for practice.

These are considered to be the integral components of developing and maintaining a portfolio. They shift the balance of maintaining a portfolio from the relatively passive exercise of describing to one that is interactive. It is the activities of continually recording, reviewing, reflecting and demonstrating that in portfolio learning facilitates self-awareness, personal growth and professional development.

While some of your entries will be a factual record of events, an essential aspect will be working with entries and making sense of what you are recording. This encourages further learning and allows you to demonstrate this in practice. In nursing a useful way of doing this is to give structure to the deliberations, and Crouch (1991) and others advocate the use of critical incidents. These are significant events with negative or positive outcomes that have meaning to you or your practice. Such incidents provide a useful way of focusing on and exploring relevant issues to gain new insights.

FIGURE 12.2   How to work with a portfolio

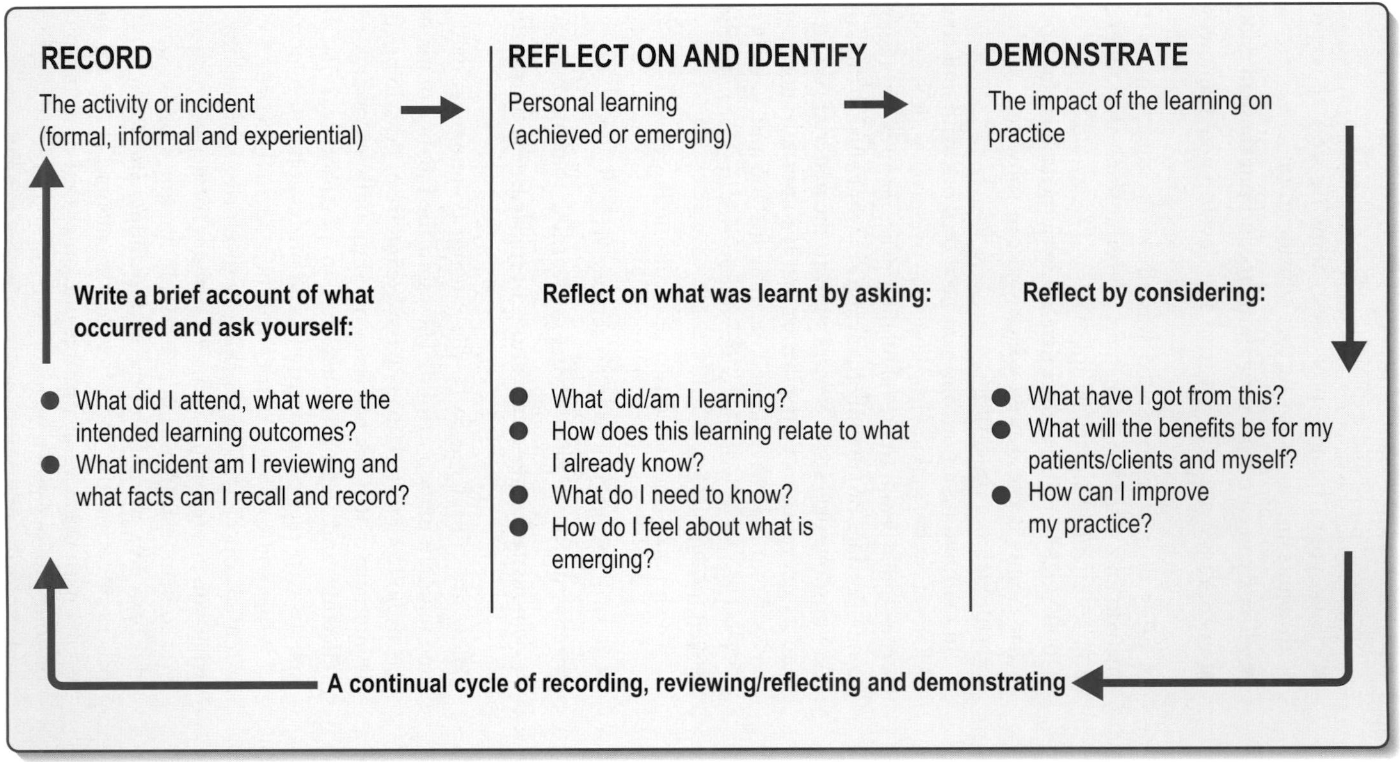

RECORD

The activity or incident (formal, informal and experiential)

Write a brief account of what occurred and ask yourself:

- What did I attend, what were the intended learning outcomes?
- What incident am I reviewing and what facts can I recall and record?

REFLECT ON AND IDENTIFY

Personal learning (achieved or emerging)

Reflect on what was learnt by asking:

- What did/am I learning?
- How does this learning relate to what I already know?
- What do I need to know?
- How do I feel about what is emerging?

DEMONSTRATE

The impact of the learning on practice

Reflect by considering:

- What have I got from this?
- What will the benefits be for my patients/clients and myself?
- How can I improve my practice?

A continual cycle of recording, reviewing/reflecting and demonstrating

BOX 12.1	**Working with a critical incident**

Identify a recent incident or experience that had significance for you, and ask yourself:

1.1   What happened?

1.2   Who was involved?

1.3   What was the outcome?

2.1   What did I feel?

2.2   What did I learn?

2.3   What would I do differently?

3.1   What have I learned from reflecting on this incident?

3.2   How will this learning impact on my practice?

In the first set of questions you are reviewing the factual events of the incident or experience and your responses can be recorded in your portfolio to allow you to work with them. In the second set of questions you are asked to engage with your feelings, as this is an integral part of helping you make sense of your learning. In the third set of questions you are asked to stand back, as it were, to consider the impact of this critical exposure that may result in changes to your practice.

Such inquiry requires a positive clinical culture that acknowledges that on many occasions we do get things right and that our patients/clients are satisfied, hence the need for identifying positive experiences as well as the negative ones. We need to know why some things go well and others less so, in order to appreciate the experience and make discerning judgements in practice. In this way we learn from our mistakes and prevent ourselves from repeating them.

Working with your entries:

■ Allow yourself adequate time

■ Let your ideas flow

■ Be honest and genuine in your recordings

■ Acknowledge when something is difficult

■ Ask yourself critical questions about what is emerging

■ Be creative and allow yourself to think differently

■ Don't confine yourself to one view

■ Seek help when it is required

As discussed previously, the portfolio is a confidential document and this remains true whether you select information for a 'personal, professional profile', share aspects with your peers, your mentor or in class, or draw on your experiences for written assignments. What is becoming evident is that, increasingly, nursing courses require that portfolios are assessed.

ASSESSING PORTFOLIOS

There is little doubt that assessing portfolios is a contentious subject as assessors and teachers grapple with ways of objectively assessing reflective work. As reflective writing includes the interpretation of feelings and personal analysis of meaningful events, this makes this part of the portfolio difficult to assess. Another complication is that a portfolio demonstrates continuing learning and is not a summative product that is readily measurable.

Other issues that make assessing portfolios difficult are that assessment requires making a judgement or grading material against preset criteria (see Chapter 7). In the case of portfolios within nursing, this includes the evaluation of the profiling element for professional accreditation or marking of course work.

It is therefore important for those involved to recognize that identifying assessment criteria for marking may affect portfolio learning and, as a consequence, the portfolio that develops. This could become more of an issue should an accrediting body seek to dictate the format and content of portfolios. The NMC has prepared flexible guidelines concerning what should be recorded, while other regulatory bodies are more prescriptive.

At present there is limited empirical evidence for making a strong case for or against assessing portfolios. Wong et al (1995) have identified difficulties in assessing levels of reflection from journals and have encountered problems in applying quantitative criteria to qualitative writing. Sumsion and Fleet (1996) have the view that current academic rating scales may be unsuitable for unravelling the complexities of reflective accounts.

However, we cannot leave it there and say categorically that portfolios can't, or shouldn't be, assessed because we know they are and because portfolios have become a significant force in continuing professional education in recent years. Pitts et al (1999, p. 517) have shown that assessing portfolios is challenging and report that 'trained assessors can only achieve a fair degree of agreement (inter-rater reliability) when judging portfolios against agreed criteria'. Others, such as Moon (1999), note that portfolios are increasingly used as evidence of reflection and suggest that teachers and programme developers should be obliged to consider appropriate assessment methods.

The following discussion and examples are offered to involve you in reflecting on the issues that assessing portfolios raises. Whether you are a student beginning your nursing career or a teacher assessing portfolio work, you are part of the assessment process. What becomes apparent in exploring the idea of assessing portfolios is that we need to think creatively about assessment methods and not rely on traditional approaches. What are required are assessments that wrestle with the complexities of subjective, narrative accounts as part of a continual cycle of learning and reflection (Greenhalgh and Hurwitz 1999; see Chapter 2).

Some researchers recommend a structure for portfolios that helps make assessment a more objective process. In their study, Challis et al (1997) link portfolio learning to the completion of a learning cycle as discussed in Chapter 2. The sample was asked to identify their learning needs and plan appropriate activities to meet these needs. The resulting portfolios included a needs analysis, an action plan and evidence that needs had been met and new learning applied to practice. Providing a framework requires an understanding of the learning process with the identification of clear aims and learning outcomes that are linked to appropriate educational activities.

A structured approach to assessing portfolios requires evidence of:

- the relationship between the aims, the outcomes and the action plan
- connections between experiences
- reflection and how this was undertaken
- knowledge management
- personal and professional development
- relating new learning to practice and the impact of learning on patients
- identification of further learning required.

Others offer a more reflective perspective and recommend that the results of assessment 'may be used to determine the value of the journal as a method of learning and facilitating learning' (Moon 1999, p. 91). This fits well with less structured approaches where those running professional development courses provide a statement of reflective competence. This approach identifies that reflection is evident but the portfolios are not graded. In other examples, teachers may offer you their own reflective account of your work, which includes reflective questions to engage you further with your writing. This encourages further learning and involves the assessment as part of the narrative that is continually reshaped and reframed.

From the discussion of the approach to be taken, a key question emerges – 'What should assessors look for in assessing portfolios?'.

Moon (1999, p. 100) offers some general criteria that can be useful in indicating adequacy and quality. These include length, presentation and legibility, number and regularities of entries, thoroughness of reflection and developing self-awareness. However, she also draws attention to criteria that you may not have considered, including:

- evidence of creativity and critical thinking
- clarity and sound observation of events
- demonstration of analysis, evaluation and synthesis of material
- connection of the content with the programme's aims and outcomes
- evidence of working through issues and acknowledging the challenges and struggles.

What begins to emerge is that, if portfolios are to be assessed effectively, you should expect explicit criteria that relate to the purpose of developing the portfolio. Any criteria should be clearly identified for all concerned and you should be given time to plan and organize your writing and to make sense of the process. Any assessment should also include preparation of students, practitioners and assessors who are involved in all aspects of identifying and testing criteria. Assessor preparation should focus on encouraging inter-rater reliability while the students' preparation should involve strategies that encourage reflection and self-assessment (Chapter 11).

SELF-ASSESSMENT

Self-assessment is an important part of portfolio learning and it is therefore essential that this aspect is included within the assessment approach. This allows you to consider the role that you have in assessing your work. This also ensures that reflection continues and that you have ownership of how your work achieves the purpose required. In making a self-assessment of your work you may like to consider (see Chapter 2):

- How do I show that I have analysed and reflected upon my key learning experiences, both formally and experientially?
- What significant learning resources have I identified and developed?
- What evidence do I offer for my personal and professional development?
- How do I demonstrate that the material is:
  - acceptable, accessible, appropriate, authentic
  - balanced, beneficial, broad
  - clear, coherent, consistent, continuing, current?

- How do I demonstrate that I have developed or changed?
- What evidence do I offer to show that the insights I have gained have changed my practice?
- How do I show that I am aware of the need for further learning?

The assessment principles listed in Box 12.2 are a useful guide.

BOX 12.2	*Assessing portfolios – the principles*

- Everyone involved is clear about the criteria for assessment
- The purpose of developing the portfolio should be reflected in the assessment rationale and criteria
- Assessment criteria and grading systems should be flexible
- Assessment should encourage further learning for both students and teachers
- Assessment should include a self-assessment component that can be documented in the developing portfolio
- Preparation should include students, practitioners and assessors in identifying and testing criteria

CONCLUSION

Developing a portfolio can help you reflect and give you time to catch up with yourself in order 'to take stock, to make sense of what has happened or share other people's ideas on the experience' (Boud et al 1985, p. 8). Working with your portfolio can also help you gain a clearer sense of knowing who you are and what you are doing – allowing you to value your uniqueness and personal contribution to the health care team.

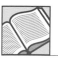

CHAPTER RESOURCES

REFERENCES

Boud D, Keogh R, Walker D 1985 Reflection: turning experience into learning. Kogan Page, London
Brown R 1995 Portfolio development and profiling for nurses, 2nd edn. Quay Books, Salisbury
Challis M, Mathers NJ, Howe AC, Field NJ 1997 Portfolio-based learning: continuing medical education for general practitioners – a mid-point evaluation. Medical Education 31: 22–26
Crouch S 1991 Critical incident analysis. Nursing 4: 30–31

Dewing J 1990 Reflective practice. Senior Nurse 10: 26–28
Gibbs G 1992 Improving the quality of student learning. Technical and
    Educational Services, Bristol
Greenhalgh T, Hurwitz B 1999 Why study narrative? British Medical Journal
    318: 48–50
Hull C, Redfern L 1996 Profiles and portfolios for nurses and midwives.
    Macmillan, London
Johns C 2000 Becoming a reflective practitioner. A reflective and holistic
    approach to clinical nursing, practice development and clinical supervision.
    Blackwell Science, Oxford
Moon J 1999 Learning journals. A handbook for academics, students and
    professional development. Kogan Page, London
Morton-Cooper A, Palmer A 2000 Mentoring, preceptorship and clinical
    supervision: a guide to professional support roles in clinical practice, 2nd edn.
    Blackwell Science, Oxford
Nursing and Midwifery Council 2001 The PREP Handbook. NMC, London
Palmer A 1993 *Nursing Times* open learning programme: an investigation in
    collaboration and design. Annals of Community Education 6: 259–272
Palmer A 2000 Freedom to learn – freedom to be: learning, reflecting and
    supporting in practice. In: Humphris D, Masterson A (eds) Developing new
    clinical roles: a guide for health professionals. Harcourt Health Sciences,
    London
Payne D 1999 UKCC threatens sanctions over PREP requirements. Nursing
    Times 95(9): 7
Pietroni R, Millard L 1996 Portfolio based learning. In: Hasler J, Pendleton D
    (eds) Professional development in general practice. Open University Press,
    Buckingham
Pitts J, Coles C, Thomas P 1999 Educational portfolios in the assessment of
    general practice trainers: reliability of assessors. Medical Education 33:
    515–520
Routledge J, Willson M, McArthur M et al 1997 Reflection on the development
    of a reflective assessment. Medical Teacher 19: 122–128
Royal College of Nursing 1990 Professional portfolios. RCN, London
Sumsion J, Fleet A 1996 Reflection: can we assess it? Should we assess it?
    Assessment and Evaluation in Higher Education 21: 121–130
Vousdon M 2000 Wake up, wise up. Nursing Times 96(8): 28–29
Wilkin M Undated. Introducing the professional development portfolio into
    your school. Essex Advisory & Inspection Service, Essex
Wong FKY, Kember D, Chung LYE, Yan L 1995 Assessing the level of
    student reflection from reflective journals. Journal of Advanced Nursing
    22: 48–57

Further reading

General Osteopathic Council 1997 The professional profile and
portfolio – standardising self-regulation. General Osteopathic
Council, London

McGrowther J 1995 Profiles, portfolios and how to build them.
Scutari Press, London

Munton R 1995 Developing your personal professional profile.
Mental Health Nursing 15: 8–10

Nursing and Midwifery Council 2001 Supporting nurses and
midwives through lifelong learning. NMC, London

Rich A, Parker D 1995 Reflection and critical incident analysis: ethical and moral implications of their use within nursing and midwifery education. Journal of Advanced Nursing 22: 1050–1057

Tsang NM 1998 Re-examining reflection – a common issue of professional concern in social work, teacher and nursing education. Journal of Interprofessional Care 12: 21–31

13 Advanced writing skills and accreditation of experiential learning

Elizabeth A Girot

INTRODUCTION

This chapter aims to develop your understanding of how to think and write reflectively within an academic framework. Chapter 11 explored the development of thinking and writing reflectively to help you study. Although the assessment of reflection is not without its difficulties (Burns and Bulman 2000), once you have begun to use reflection to help you learn from your experiences, you may wish to translate those thoughts or writings into a format that can be accredited for academia. Many educational programmes now recognize the value of reflection for practice and encourage the use of reflective writing in the course assignments. Alternatively, you may wish to claim academic recognition for your practice through presenting a claim for accreditation for your experience (accreditation of experiential learning; AEL) and be required to document your practice achievements in an academic way. An overview of the AEL system will be presented, followed by some examples of writing reflectively for academia, whatever the goal.

A number of recent reports commissioned by nursing and midwifery's statutory body (UKCC 1999a) and the Department of Health (1999, 2000) have recommended a more flexible approach to education and training, particularly for entry to preregistration nursing and midwifery programmes with the introduction of AEL. Although in the past AEL has been available to many candidates within the university system, within nursing and midwifery it has been available only to qualified practitioners. Those experienced practitioners with a wealth of expertise and years of non-accredited study have been able to seek exemption from parts of their programme of study if they can provide evidence of prior learning. This does, however, mean that they have had to identify what they have learned from their experience and articulate it in such a way as to demonstrate thinking at a particular academic level.

Following acceptance of the recommendations from the above reports (Department of Health 1999, UKCC 1999a), it should be possible for those with prior qualifications, e.g. National Vocational Qualifications (NVQs)/Scottish Vocational Qualifications (SVQs) and/or prior experience to present evidence of a non-standard nature to gain entry into and/or exemption from some of the units of study within a preregistration programme, as long as it is still relevant and current (see below). For those with prior clinical experience, this is a major change in policy. It means that those with qualifications within the practice area will not need to repeat work in which they are already deemed to be competent and will be able to seek exemption from part of their programme should they wish to apply for professional preparation. Practice within the clinical area should therefore be seen much more as a continuum and development for each individual. Ultimately, it is hoped that this new approach will attract more recruits with a wider range of skills and abilities into the profession. It is important that you should understand what is required if you wish to make such a claim.

If you are unfamiliar with the AEL system, Box 13.1 provides a simple definition:

BOX 13.1

Accreditation of experiential learning refers to the process of identification, assessment and formal acknowledgement of prior learning and achievement. 'It is the achievement of learning or the outcomes of that learning and not just the experience of the activities alone that is being accredited' (Quality Assurance Agency 2004, p. 3).

This learning may take many forms, including professional work experience, short non-assessed courses and general life experiences. However, you need to translate this experience into evidence. This evidence needs to relate to and be comparable with an existing programme of study so that you can be exempt from that part of the programme. Most programmes of study in the UK are now modularized, i.e. they are packaged up into distinct units of study. This makes the presentation of evidence a much more manageable activity for you. The modules will have clearly expressed learning outcomes or goals to be achieved and these will also be written at a particular academic level based on a typical 3-year degree programme at university.

Having this evidence accredited is only of value if you wish to follow a particular academic programme, towards a recognized award, at a particular higher education establishment. In other words, AEL claims are only of value at the particular academic institution from which you are seeking a specific award. It is generally not possible to make a claim at one institution and have it accepted at another institution. Although there may be some locally accepted arrangements, as a rule, you must make the claim at the particular institution from which you are seeking the award. You will also see the term 'accreditation of learning' (AL). This is the gaining of academic credit for the learning that is achieved from a formally taught course that has been assessed and certificated. Some nursing and midwifery departments have produced a tariff list, which shows how much credit specific courses can attract. This is generally used when transferring actual credit from one university to another.

In summary, AEL is a system by which you can gain non-standard access to or exemption from, parts of a programme of study. It should be possible now to gain non-standard entry to a programme of study and exemption from parts of preregistration programmes through the production of acceptable evidence. This may be achieved either through a system of AL (previously certificated courses) or from your past experience (through AEL). Whatever recognition you are seeking it is important to be clear that it is your prior learning that is valued and it can also contribute to and extend your learning through your ongoing studies.

THE AEL PROCESS

The AEL process can be divided into several distinct stages, which are a guide to the practitioner when claiming credit. Every institution will have its own guide or handbook for using AEL within that particular organization. Do enquire at the institution of your choice before embarking on compiling your evidence. The following is offered as a general guide only.

Stage 1: Decide on your programme of study

First, as a postqualifying nurse or midwife, you need to decide which overall programme of study you wish to follow and, subsequently, which modules you are required to complete to gain your award. Each institution will have its own distinct diploma and degree programmes, so do make sure you are clear about what is on offer and why you might be interested in that particular award. Some are specialist-focused, others are more generic. Some are very flexible and others not so. You will be required to match your experience to date against this range of individual modules and their learning outcomes.

Alternatively, as an assistant practitioner, you may have been practising within a healthcare setting for some years and, as recommended by Peach (UKCC 1999a) and the Department of Health (1999), wish to present evidence of this as access to a formalized education programme towards professional registration. You may also be able to seek exemption from parts of this programme during the first year of study. Therefore, you need to decide which programme you are interested in and at which institution. If possible, look at programme plans from several institutions and match these with your previous and current experience so that you get a more continuous process of learning. Always obtain as much information as possible, both about the programmes on offer and whether it is possible to make an AEL claim.

Stage 2: Identifying and reviewing experiences

Although you may have considerable life and/or work experience, it is not the time in practice or experience that counts in AEL but evidence of the learning that has been achieved. After all, we all know practitioners who have been practising for many years but who have not actually progressed in the quality of their practice since their first weeks of starting. Others, however, have kept themselves up to date with current developments, read widely and tried to improve their standards of care.

To present the evidence of your achievements, therefore, you need to select which prior experiences can be matched to specific learning outcomes within your chosen programme of study. To do this you need to focus clearly on experiences that have led to valuable learning. While a claim for academic credit must be current, i.e. within approximately the last 5 years, experience prior to this will be considered if you can show how you have updated older learning and applied it to your practice.

Stage 3: Identifying learning achievements

When you have identified some of your experiences that can be used for the purpose of either gaining access to a programme of study or exemption from some parts of that programme, you need to clarify what you have learned. One way of achieving this is to reflect on your experience and make some sense of it, relevant to the expected learning outcomes of the module or unit of study you are matching it against. If you look back to Chapter 11, the different frameworks that are presented may help you to break down your experiences into the different types of learning you have achieved. As you can see from Chapter 11, merely telling the story is not in itself true reflection, you need to try to identify aspects of your experience that you can make sense of in relation to your present and future practice. Asking yourself the 'So what' question at the different parts of your 'story' should help you to analyse your experience; the 'Now what' question will then help you apply what you have experienced to your learning and identify a way forward for future practice. It was pointed out in Chapter 11 that having someone with you when you ask these questions might help you to tease out the relevant meaning the different parts of your 'story' had for you.

Learning from both personal and professional achievement can be considered as long as the learning has relevance to the specific learning outcomes identified. It may be helpful to group together achievements under common headings, so you can compile your evidence in a comprehensive and coherent way. As in any academic piece of work, organizing your work in a structured and logical manner is crucial to the achievement of a good mark. The examiner should be able to read your work and know that you have a clear idea of its meaning in relation to the part of the programme against which you are seeking exemption.

Stage 4: Matching the learning achievements against the modular learning outcomes

To be considered for accreditation, your AEL claim must contain prior learning that meets the following requirements:

■ **Comparability**: the evidence you produce should match the learning outcomes of a specific module(s) approved by the university for the award sought. Not only should the type of learning match but the level of learning should also be consistent with the academic level of the learning outcomes expressed. Sometimes it is possible to undertake some taught modules or units of study first before making such a claim. In this way, you will be able to recognize levels of learning and how to structure your work in such a way that makes the most of your effort. Finding your way into the 'system' through some regular contact with the university will certainly help you when you come to develop your claim for exemption, when you are forced to work more on your own with some help from an AEL advisor.

■ **Currency**: the evidence you produce should demonstrate that the learning you have achieved is in keeping with expectations of knowledge current in the area of expertise required. Normally, evidence that is presented should be no more than 5 years old. That is, your experience may be much older than this but your reading and support for your learning should be recent. The evidence should be sufficient in amount and this will vary within and across the different universities. Do ask how much you are expected to produce; often it is the more succinct and focused work that provides the best of evidence.

■ **Authenticity**: the evidence you produce should demonstrate that you completed the work yourself.

There may be a limit to the amount of AEL you can be exempted from in any one programme. Each institution has its own limit. However, you can understand that, if you were to seek exemption from 90% of an award, it would be difficult for the institution to give its name to that award, especially if you undertook most of the work at other institutions. Some organizations limit the amount of AEL you can use to gain an award to two-thirds of the programme; others limit the amount to less.

The evidence will be scrutinized with the same rigour required of those examining standard assignments with the institution. After all, the way candidates' work is handled within the university must be consistent across the different programmes, whether the work is produced for AEL or for standard assignment work.

Types of evidence that you may like to consider

Presentation of your learning achievements may be made in a variety of ways and you must be guided by the requirements of the institution to which you are making your claim.

■ Teaching package: implemented and evaluated

■ Innovations in practice, e.g. introduction of a change in practice, standard setting

■ Practical evidence: care plans, information leaflets

■ Analysis of a clinical incident

■ Case studies

■ Reports

■ Budgets

■ Audio/video tapes

■ Essay/project

■ Evidence of peer review, appraisal or inspection processes

■ Interview

- Alternatively, if you have recently completed a programme of study that has not been academically accredited, it may be appropriate to complete the actual module assignment

- Assessment of professional competence. Sometimes there is little or no formal 'input' but a considerable amount of assessment by 'internal or external verifiers' (e.g. for NVQs). For these, you will need to provide a copy of your certificate and a letter describing the type and frequency of assessment, evidence submitted and range indicators, e.g. City & Guilds Assessor Awards. In addition, you will need to accompany your submission with a written commentary to demonstrate equivalence of learning outcomes to those modules or units you are specifically claiming against. In this way, you can demonstrate the appropriate academic quality.

Academic portfolio

Where you need to present evidence of learning from a variety of experiences, you can do this through the development of an academic portfolio (Chapter 12). An academic portfolio may have two distinct parts:

- An accredited learning section, which provides evidence of formal learning that has already been accredited and certificated by a recognized higher education institution or assessed by recognized agencies and for which you are now seeking university credit

- An experiential learning section providing evidence of your learning from experience.

It is hoped that you may have some evidence in both sections.

BOX 13.2

Accredited learning section

In this section, you will need to identify:

- Which module or unit of the programme you are seeking exemption from on the basis of your existing credit

- Copies of any relevant certificates and any associated credit transcripts

- For non-credit-rated programmes, a copy of the associated syllabus, programme of study, length of study, number and length of assignments and assessment criteria used will need to be presented

- A copy of relevant assignments together with tutor feedback.

Experiential learning section

In this section, you will need to identify:

- Which module or unit of the programme you are seeking exemption from on the basis of your experience

■ The experiences you have had that have led to the learning evidenced. This must be accompanied by a written commentary to support the appropriate academic level of the unit. The learning outcomes of the matched module or unit you are interested in seeking exemption from must be presented, with the appropriate evidence alongside.

Stage 5: Summarizing the AEL claim

To help you in the submission of your AEL claim, each institution that offers this facility should have a key person, usually called an AEL co-ordinator, to give you advice as to how your evidence should be presented. Most institutions have a handbook or document that shows clearly how the evidence should be presented. Additionally, some institutions offer workshops or individual support for the submission of your claim and there is usually a fee required for your submission to be considered.

Once you have developed your academic portfolio and presented your evidence against a particular module or unit of study, you need to summarize your claim and submit this summary along with the main body of your claim. This acts as an aid to assessment of your AEL claim and demonstrates clearly how your learning experiences have led to a coherent learning achievement. The actual layout will vary according to the different institutions. You must be guided by your AEL advisor.

LEVELS OF LEARNING

The process of learning within academic programmes in institutions of higher education progresses through different levels of learning. Various frameworks have been used to guide this learning but essentially there is a hierarchy of educational development that achievement can be measured against. Some of these frameworks are as follows.

Steinaker and Bell's (1979) experiential taxonomy of achievement in practice:

■ **Exposure:** consciousness of an experience – having the skill demonstrated
■ **Participation:** deciding to become part of an experience – practice in the activity
■ **Identification:** union of the learner with what is to be learned – competency in achievement of the skill

- **Internalization:** experience continues to influence lifestyle – mastery of the activity
- **Dissemination:** attempt to influence others, e.g. through teaching.

This hierarchy can guide you to articulating different levels of practical achievement, which progress through both the *doing* of the practice as well as the *thinking* behind what you are doing. Sometimes in an academic paper it is difficult to find ways to articulate higher levels of practice when, for example, you are concerned with doing the practice safely. Translating this into academic writing may initially cause you some difficulty.

Alternatively, Bloom (1956) formulated a hierarchy of levels in each of the three areas of learning as follows:

- knowledge domain (cognitive)
- skills domain (psychomotor)
- attitudes domain (affective).

Until recently, most academic programmes have been loosely based on Bloom's cognitive hierarchy, although some newer frameworks, e.g. that of the Southern England Consortium for Credit Accumulation and Transfer (SECC 2003), have adapted these to include the practice skills and generic transferable skills as well as the cognitive skills.

Most university degree programmes follow a developmental structure, moving from lower-order skills equivalent to the first year of a higher education degree towards the higher-order skills in the final year of a degree. The different levels indicate a progressive 'level of demand, complexity, depth of study and student autonomy' (SECC 2003, p. 5). Although there are a number of level descriptors used throughout the UK, the SECC level descriptors are one of the most widely used in higher education.

However, not all descriptors are relevant to all degrees, or all modules of study, although most are relevant to most units of study (Gosling and Moon 2002). Therefore you will find that the marking guidelines for assignments in your own programme of study may have specific descriptors picked out of the framework against which your work will be marked and these will relate to the expectations of that unit of study. These level descriptors will also act as a guide to your writing when making your AEL claim. Unlike Bloom (1956), SECC makes explicit the expectations of each level of any higher education programme in relation to each of the different skills.

Each university will have its own expectations of the different levels articulated so that you can be guided when presenting your written commentary, linked to the matched module or unit outcomes.

Whatever the academic level, you must present your evidence supported by relevant and current literature. All university institutions will require you to follow a specific system of referencing; although many now advocate the Harvard system of referencing (see Chapter 10 for further information on this system).

Summary of the AEL process

In summary, therefore, AEL is a way of gaining non-standard entry to a particular programme of your choice, or exemption from some part of that programme towards the achievement of an award. Each higher education institution has its own process governed by its own rules and regulations. You must seek guidance from the AEL co-ordinator before embarking on this process of compiling a claim so that you are absolutely clear as to what is expected of you. I have attempted to present a general framework of the process expected from you in most institutions, the different types of evidence that you can use and the different levels of learning that can help you articulate your learning at the appropriate academic level. I believe it would be helpful at this point to present some examples of how to write reflectively for academia, especially if you have been used to producing third-person academic writing.

WRITING REFLECTIVELY FOR ACADEMIA

Whatever the reason, if you need to translate your reflective writing and thought processes into the rigour of an academic assignment, similar rules apply to both first-person reflective writing and third-person academic writing. However, rather than write in the third person, as most academic programmes encourage, the reflective approach encourages you to maintain a first-person reflective style of writing while at the same time supporting your thoughts and feelings with reference to the literature and research.

It is useful to think of writing in the first person as a great privilege. You need to think carefully when using this approach, so as not to use it as a chatty, letter-writing activity where it is easy to 'tell your story'. As you saw in Chapter 11, telling your story is only one small part of the reflective process. As Rolfe et al acknowledge (2001, p, 42), reflective writing involves engaging in and completing the reflective cycle to learn from the experience while at the same time recognizing the difficulties involved in exposing self in this approach. I often ask students to look at themselves from above or outside themselves when engaging in their reflective analysis. It is almost like trying to justify and rationalize what they did and why they did it, supporting their justification with evidence from the literature. As you have probably only had experience of writing in the first person when engaging in friendly chat, e.g. letter writing, it is easy to get caught in the trap of purely descriptive passages along the lines of 'You'll never guess what happened to me the other day . . .' However, as has already been explained, friendly chat and purely descriptive story telling are unacceptable as evidence against academic claims or as evidence for academic assignments. Considering it a privilege to write in the first person may allow you to use it with caution in as much as having to justify your actions.

Examples of reflective writing are becoming more evident in the literature (e.g. Burns and Bulman 2000) and it is important that, before writing your reflective academic assignment, you read a range of examples to give you an idea of best practice. Some of my own students have written reflective assignments to demonstrate, on reflection, how they went about planning and justifying a particular approach to the organization of a teaching session. As a result of their own developments, I would like to share excerpts from their reflective writing. All students were undertaking a postqualifying course on teaching and assessing in practice, level 3 (degree level) and these excerpts mostly represent their first attempt at such writing. Nevertheless, there are some insightful examples of their critical reflection.

One student, Jane, clarified for herself the value of reflection for her own learning. She recognized how easy it is to gain experience from her work but not necessarily to have learned from it.

CASE STUDY   **Jane**

Reflective practice pushes the 'learning from experience' to its ultimate limit by facilitating the process of change. . . . Street (1991) identifies that learning does not always develop from experience. It is therefore vital that the reflective process is an integral part of any nurse practitioner role, both as clinician and as teacher or assessor in the clinical area. . . . Through the process of reflection an attempt has been made to link teaching and assessing theory to practice, thereby attempting to understand how those areas of shortfall might be improved. Reflection also offers the opportunity to explore the reason for shortfalls in performance, and it can offer ideas as to how to improve performance.

Here Jane is justifying to herself the importance of reflection and identifying not only what she might gain from this reflection – facilitating the process of change – but also recognizing that it is a process and not simply story-telling.

Jane begins her reflection. She remembers well her feelings on arrival at the planned session and how that influenced her approach. She decided to reflect on her approach to questioning as a method of teaching and could rationally think about the merits and problems of different approaches to questioning. However, her anxiety when faced with a number of experienced practitioners adversely affected her performance.

CASE STUDY

Jane

The lesson plan acknowledged the need to keep active connection with the audience; a group of eight professionals with a wide range of experiences in health promotion. During the assessment of the learners' prior knowledge and needs it had been identified by the group that interaction throughout the session was desirable. I decided that questions would facilitate that interaction, particularly at the start of the session.

As the session progressed I could feel anxiety building in my body. I had arrived at the venue aware that I was about to deliver the topic of Mental Health Promotion to a group of highly experienced professionals, some of whom had careers spanning many facets of health and education. They were mature, articulate and bright.

When I arrived in the room I felt extremely nervous. I felt vulnerable and insecure despite the warm welcome and the assistance to place the equipment and furniture in appropriate places. At times I felt detached from my own body as if observing the whole event from an aerial position. My movements became somewhat mechanical. I could feel myself over-compensating, being overly happy and chatty.

As the teaching session commenced I was unable to relax despite feeling safe and welcomed. I began the session and could sense a speed of speech in my voice and I continued to feel detached from myself. The early questions designed to allow audience participation were delivered in a rhetorical manner, answered by myself with the content of the session quickly resumed with speed and wilfulness. I knew this was not good teaching practice but could not change the pattern.

Although Jane was a qualified teacher, it was clear from her reflection that she was adversely influenced by the potentially powerful effect of her audience. It is somewhat reassuring to hear Jane articulate her feelings and recognize this effect and how she began to overcome her feelings:

CASE STUDY

Jane

As time developed, and audience members politely intercepted my talk to ask questions, this had the effect of creating a positive change in my anxiety levels. I became more relaxed into the session and could feel myself letting go of the need to be the perfect fount of knowledge. After ten minutes I was able to ask a question and allow time for a response. I started to enjoy the session and the audience appeared less frustrated. On reflection, my anxiety was probably born out of a feeling of insecurity about my professional ability, and a feeling of intimidation being surrounded by a group of experienced professionals.

She then goes on to consider in more depth the importance of questioning and the different types of question that can be used.

Another student, Marcia, sought to justify teaching away from her practice area for her formal assessment of the course.

CASE STUDY   **Marcia**

When considering planning this session, I actively rejected the notion of undertaking it within my own area of clinical practice. I am a staff nurse working within ophthalmic trauma in a teaching hospital, where all nursing staff are qualified and the majority also hold a post-basic qualification. . . . I felt threatened about practising the skill of formal teaching, which is new to me, with colleagues whose speciality knowledge base is high. Quinn (1995) suggests that by taking on the role of teacher you may be inferring that you have more knowledge than your learner. On reflection, I feel that the view of the teacher in adult learning as more of a guide and facilitator is more appropriate (Knowles 1990), as this acknowledges the value of the learner's experience.

As you can see from this example, Marcia openly expresses her feelings about the situation and begins to analyse it and support her thoughts with current literature. The process is no less rigorous than that used in the third-person, impersonal academic style of writing, yet it comes alive and has meaning for the individual concerned and direct relevance to her own practice. Those reading it also gain by recognizing similar feelings and justification for moving in different directions. Like Jane, Marcia felt threatened but actively took steps to overcome as much of that threat as possible.

CASE STUDY   **Marcia**

I contacted the sister prior to the session to ask what topic area they would like me to cover. In consultation with her staff she identified assessment and record keeping. . . . I felt this was important as the idea of andragogy, which will be discussed in more depth later, places the learners as central in identifying learning needs (Nielson 1992). It was interesting that I would have selected a topic related to disease or trauma of the eye. Kenworthy and Nicklin (1988) counsel against selecting pet topics that may not be of value. In my experience both of these points proved relevant as feedback from both the group and facilitator confirmed that the subject had met their learning needs and I would certainly use this strategy for a similar session.

Here again, the student enters into dialogue with herself. She recognizes the need as teacher to enable the students to identify their own learning needs. She also recognizes that, if given the choice herself, she would have picked her own pet subject, quite different from that chosen by the student group and not so appropriate. She analyses the issues and examines alternatives, supporting her choices with current literature.

Marcia continues in her reflective evaluation of her teaching.

CASE STUDY   **Marcia**

The use of lectures is suggested to be the antithesis of student-centred learning, and certainly Harvey and Vaughan (1990) found in a study that student nurses did not have a positive reaction to them, although I would suggest that this may be a reflection of their operational definition of a lecture as solely a one-way communication. I felt that the lecture/discussion was of value and had a place in an andragogical approach, a view shared by Jones (1990); not, as O'Kell (1988) implies, due to nurses adopting a passive role, but as an appropriate way of introducing new information (Knowles 1990). I also acknowledge that I selected a lecture as a strategy in part because I felt more comfortable with it as I had more control. It is interesting that Dux (1989) noted the popularity of lectures with nurse teachers, although the study does not identify why. I feel that I would use the strategy of a lecture/discussion through the fictional patient. I feel that the amount of discussion was in part due to the group rather than my teaching skill. Perhaps this could be achieved through more use of questioning (Quinn 1995).

Here again, Marcia explores her own thoughts and feelings about what she did and analyses the various issues, accepting and rejecting aspects of the literature in support of her own situation. Overall, however, she consistently explores the learning she has achieved from the various activities and I suspect will continue her exploration as she develops her skills as a facilitator of learning.

Following an analysis of the different types of questioning, Jane, too, finds a way forwards for herself.

CASE STUDY   **Jane**

In analysing and reflecting on my own poor questioning skills I would suggest that my anxiety resulted in a need to answer the questions myself because of a lack of confidence to be able to cope with any answers which might challenge my knowledge. I believe that if I had felt more confident this would have resulted in a relaxed style of teaching with the ability to become vulnerable if exposed as not knowledgeable. Reece and Walker (1995) confirm this view and advocate the need to develop confidence in both subject matter and preparation of material in order to reduce any lack of confidence. They believe that such confidence leads to more creative teaching skills being used by the teacher, and enables greater interaction by the learners. Creative use of question strategy could include use of open and closed questions, use of body language and non-verbal cues to evoke answers and awareness of the answering needs and voice of all members of the audience.

Since I believe that my preparation for the teaching session was of a high standard, I have reflected on an action plan that I might implement in order to avoid the misuse of questioning skills in the future – in particular the inappropriate use of rhetorical questions. In future I would try to recognize the signs of anxiety within myself prior to the start of a teaching session and try to alleviate that stress by admitting to the audience of my state. I would try to introduce humour if possible as a means of breaking the ice.

I believe that anxiety in the teaching role will occur from time to time, particularly in more formal presentations, and since I believe that my thorough preparation and topic knowledge helped me to harness the anxiety felt on this particular session, then I would always arrive well prepared in the future.

In summary, therefore, Jane begins by being overcome by her anxiety in spite of careful preparation for her session. She justifies why she has chosen the use of questioning as a teaching method and analyses how she performed. As she does so, she is looking at her own performance as if detached from herself in order to present some objective view of her analysis. She then uses the literature to support how she might overcome her lack of skilled performance in the future – the 'now what' of Driscoll's (1994) framework.

Another student, Margaret, a health visitor, reflects on her teaching session with a preregistration student in the community.

CASE STUDY

Margaret

On reflection I am pleased with the way I dealt with this session. I was able to bring the teaching material down to an appropriate level for this student by revising some basic theory before moving on to the task in hand. Looking back I realize that this was an example of 'reflection-in-action' (Schon 1991), i.e. I was able to develop variations according to my on-the-spot understanding of the problems of this student. I would like to suggest, however, that while this adaptation of teaching material was possible in a one-to-one teaching session, it would be far more difficult to achieve were I to try to listen and respond to the problems of individual students if I were to undertake this teaching session with a large group of students.

As with Marcia and Jane, Margaret looks back on her experience and begins to link theory with practice. She actively analyses her teaching session in relation to this individual learner as well as recognizing the difficulties in adapting her suggestions for a larger group of students. In addition, she refers to 'reflection-in-action' (Schon 1991), i.e. thinking on your feet and adapting your activities as you are doing them. As a professional nurse or midwife, you will be reflecting-in-action all the time and adapting your care to suit individual needs. However, as Margaret has recognized, it is important to articulate this and identify how you are making your decisions.

As with the previous two students, Margaret recognizes the value of Knowles's (1990) work and its application to her own teaching in the community.

CASE STUDY

Margaret

Knowles (1990) suggests that the teaching–learning transaction is a mutual responsibility between teacher and student, a view which I strongly support. I feel that student responsibility is of particular relevance in the nursing profession as preparation for the ongoing learning experiences after qualification when the practitioner must ensure she is up to date with relevant research (UKCC 1992). Self-directed learning is likely to become even more important as cash-starved Trusts, coupled with a shortage of available courses, place responsibility for updating knowledge squarely on the shoulders of the practitioner.

On reflection, however, the student I was teaching was very young and it may have been unreasonable to expect a student at this stage in her training to employ a way of learning that she may have had little experience of. Kenworthy and Nicklin (1988), for example, suggest that students who come into nursing straight from school, as she had, may have well-established concepts of teacher-led learning.

I cannot therefore relinquish all the responsibility for the student's lack of prior knowledge. If independent study is viewed as capability to be developed in a student (Dressel and Thompson 1973), perhaps I did not spend enough time helping her to identify her learning needs.

While overall Margaret was pleased with the way the session had gone, she recognized a number of areas that could be improved.

CASE STUDY

Margaret

On reflection immediately after the session, however, I realized I had tried to cram too much material into one session. I had covered all the material but had achieved breadth at the expense of depth. In future I would certainly plan at least two sessions to cover this subject. . . . In relation to this it occurred to me that I did not actually know how much the student had learned at the end of the session. We read through the objectives and agreed that we had met them but I did not actually revisit the objectives by questioning the student on her newly found knowledge. Questioning at the end of the session is suggested to enhance the retention of lecture material (Bligh 1972), and I think in future sessions of this nature I would offer a brief quiz or self-assessment test both to enhance memory and to provide feedback.

I wonder now if one reason that I did not fully revisit the objectives as I had intended to was a 'defence mechanism' on my part. I had already felt 'let down' by her at the beginning of the session and did not wish to repeat the experience at the end, e.g. if I found she had not learned much. Why did I have this feeling of being let down? I think it was probably because I am a novice teacher and wished to perform well, as I was being assessed. . . .

This is a painful reflection because it shows that I was, as teacher, placing my needs centrally before those of the student – a concept which is in direct contradiction to the ethos of adult learning (Knowles 1990) that I profess to be aiming for in this teaching session. In future I shall have to ensure that I am on my guard against this in order that I can enable the student(s) to learn effectively.

Margaret has expressed here a truly insightful reflection. Initially, she explores the issues rather superficially. However, she then begins to express her thoughts and feelings with regard to a more in-depth analysis of the situation. She freely admits the painful experience it has been, but emerges from the reflection as having learned something positive that she can take with her to other sessions in the future.

One final student, Clare, reflects on her assessment of a student's competence putting up an intravenous infusion system. At the end of the assessment she identified that the student was neither safe nor competent in this skill and attempted to analyse the situation and justify why she felt this to be so.

CASE STUDY   **Clare**

Initially I explained to the student what I expected of her and what I would be looking for. I made it clear that I expected her to know why, the rationale, for giving the patient intravenous fluids. It was her failure to be able to answer this question that gave me an 'experience of surprise', which Schon (1991) identifies as the first stage of the reflective process. I used further questions: What is the most common reason for giving fluids to patients here? What operation did the patient have? And finally, How much can the patient drink at the moment? At which point the student was able to answer correctly. Rowntree (1987) suggests this questioning technique enables students to learn by making them think through and remember the process. On reflection I had not realized I used this technique. Reflecting in action I had felt I was using questions in an effort to draw out knowledge to link theory to practice.

We often have a 'gut feeling' that someone is not safe, but it is only when we try to articulate why this may be so that we can clarify the criteria we are using and, in turn, help the student to see exactly what is wrong with the performance.

CASE STUDY   **Clare**

I then moved the student on to the practical skill of running the fluids through a giving set. . . . How did I assess that the student was not competent? When planning the assessment I had initially set a standard to be achieved of 'safe practitioner', though Quinn (1995) argues that safety is necessary but not a sufficient condition for competence. What influenced my choice of standard?

Safety is frequently mentioned in the Steinaker and Bell (1979) stages of achievement, which is how the student was being assessed on the placement. Though her failure to provide rationale, to understand the 'why' she was doing it, would suggest she did not meet the required level. Jarvis (1985) defines competence as the successful integration of theory and practice and for the same reasons the student was not competent using this definition.

Clare's probing of her assessment delved deeper into rationalizing her judgement.

CASE STUDY **Clare**

How did I feel about this experience when it was happening (Johns 1993)? Early in the assessment I began to feel the student was not competent, how did I know so quickly? I used Benner's (1984) ideas to look at myself, the 'attention to self necessary for reflective practice' suggested by Lauterbach and Hentz-Becker (1996). Was I an 'expert' using 'intuition' to judge the situation? Benner's model seems to be related to clinical practice, but analysis of her model (Rolfe 1997) suggests it is equally relevant to the 'skill' of assessment. Rolfe (1997) discusses the use of experience of similar situations as 'paradigm cases' (p. 93), though While (1994) suggests competence is inferred from limited observations.

As you can see, Clare's style of writing is rather different from that of the other three. She follows Johns' framework of questions, of prompts to guide her reflections. This does allow the depth of thought to emerge and provides a truly analytical approach to this assessment situation.

I hope these examples will give you some idea of how to develop your reflective writing into an academic piece of work. The result offers you a truly analytical approach to your own learning. As you can see, it must be supported by current literature and, where possible, current research.

However, the above examples do not necessarily give you a feel for the whole picture in terms of structure. Overall, the structure of your assignment, or evidence presented for an AEL claim, will be the same as you are required to present for any third-person academic assignment, i.e. it must have an introduction, main body and conclusion. In addition, the main body needs to be well structured and follow logically sequenced thoughts and arguments – all that you have learned in earlier chapters, particularly Chapter 9. However, here, you are encouraged to express your feelings, just as the major writers on reflection have identified. From the above examples, the recognition of the feelings you have experienced is a major element of the learning process. It is almost like revisiting the experience for yourself, but somehow standing outside yourself and discussing the decision-making process that you were involved in when making your decisions.

As you can see from the above examples, these students thought through why they organized their teaching and assessing in the way that they did, identified the advantages, recognized the different problems, but finally came to a decision about how they presented their session given the various options available. They reasoned through the decision-making process, discounting a number of options open to them. As in third-person academic work, it is equally important here to develop and present your analysis of the process and not merely describe the situation. It is not an easy skill to achieve. While description is a part of the process, it is only one part, and it is the development of analytical thought that will represent the different academic levels. Like any academic assignment, it is important to identify what is expected from the different levels of academia in your particular institution, as they do vary slightly throughout the country.

In addition to the hierarchy of the cognitive domain, as identified by Bloom (1956), Mezirow (1981) offered a hierarchy of seven levels of reflectivity, ranging from a purely descriptive approach to gaining insightful learning to a sophisticated analytical process:

1 **Reflective:** becoming aware of a specific perception, meaning or behaviour of your own or the habits you have of seeing, thinking and acting
2 **Affective:** becoming aware of how you feel about the way you are perceiving, thinking or acting
3 **Discriminant:** assessing the efficacy of your expectations, thoughts and actions. Recognizing the reality of the contexts in which you work and identifying your relationship to the situation
4 **Judgemental:** making and becoming aware of your value judgements about your perception, thought and actions, in terms of being positive or negative
5 **Conceptual:** being conscious of your awareness and being critical of it (e.g. being critical of the concepts you use to evaluate a situation)
6 **Psychic:** recognizing in yourself the habit of making precipitant judgements about people based on limited information
7 **Theoretical:** becoming aware of the influence of underlying assumptions upon your judgement.

Powell (1989) adapted Mezirow's seven levels of reflectivity to six levels in her small study of nurses in the UK, to find out whether nurses do reflect in practice and, if so, to what level. In essence, she found that her small sample (eight nurses) demonstrated extensive but superficial levels of reflection with little critical and analytical thought. This is further supported in the UKCC's study (1999b) into the reflective activity of professional practitioners applying for re-registration. Certainly, if you wish to use your reflective practice for academic assignment work or as a contribution towards an AEL claim, these activities demand that the higher levels of reflection are used. In addition, support from the literature and research is required to justify what you have done in practice.

As recognized at the beginning of this chapter, the assessment of reflection is not without its difficulties (Burns and Bulman 2000). However, it is clear from the examples presented in this chapter that students have gained from their experiences both in terms of academic credit, but more importantly, they have begun to articulate their deep levels of learning from practice. As shown in Chapter 11, developing a learning culture within the workplace helps the team to support each other. Gaining recognition of this learning through an AEL process also encourages you as an individual to pursue your own goals.

CONCLUSION

This chapter has introduced to you the notion of thinking and writing reflectively within an academic framework. It has given you an overview of the AEL process and the different levels of academic expectations. Some examples have been offered as an illustration of how to put your writing into this academic framework. Now you need to put this together with ideas from earlier chapters on the various aspects of assignment writing. Most importantly, you should recognize that, whether using a third-person academic style of writing or a first-person reflective style, the rigour required by academia is the same.

■ Reflection for academic credit must be of the appropriate quality in relation to levels of learning.

■ If not already familiar with the academic system, you should seek advice regarding what is expected of you by the university you are attending.

■ When writing reflection at academic level 3 (degree), critical thought, analysis, synthesis and evaluation must be evident (several examples are given).

■ As with all academic work, your reflective writing for academic purposes must follow the same rules as with third-person, impersonal writing, i.e. structure and logical sequencing of ideas must be evident. Support from the literature must be no less rigorous than with other academic work.

■ Next time one of your colleagues shares their reflections with you, encourage them to analyse the situation rather than simply describe it.

Listen to what they have to say. Also, try to identify what, most of all, they have learned from the situation.

■ If you already have a clinical forum where you discuss incidents that occur in your workplace, try to look at the situations from different perspectives. Encourage everyone involved to put their own view forward. Try to act as devil's advocate! Afterwards, write the discussion in your portfolio. Try to make sense of the discussion by examining the literature to give you some substance to the discussion.

■ Compare your work with some of the above examples. Show your work to your link tutor or to a colleague with an academic background to see if they can offer any support.

 CHAPTER RESOURCES

REFERENCES

Benner P 1984 From novice to expert. Addison-Wesley, Menlo Park, CA

Bligh D 1972 What's the good of lectures? Penguin Educational, Harmondsworth

Bloom B 1956 Taxonomy of educational objectives. Handbook 1. Cognitive domain. McKay, New York

Burns S, Bulman C (eds) 2000 Reflective practice in nursing: the growth of the professional practitioner, 2nd edn. Blackwell Science, Oxford

Department of Health 1999 Making a difference: strengthening the nursing, midwifery and health visiting contribution to health and healthcare. The Stationery Office, London

Department of Health 2000 A health service of all the talents: developing the NHS workforce. The Stationery Office, London

Dressel PL, Thompson MM 1973 Independent study. Jossey-Bass, San Francisco

Driscoll J 1994 Reflective practice for practice. Senior Nurse 13: 47–50

Dux CM 1989 An investigation into whether nurse teachers take into account the individual learning styles of their students when formulating teaching strategies. Nurse Education Today 9: 186–191

Gosling D, Moon J 2002 How to use learning outcomes and assessment criteria, 2nd edn. Southern England Consortium for Credit Accumulation and Transfer, London

Harvey TJ, Vaughan J 1990 Student nurse attitudes towards different teaching/learning methods. Nurse Education Today 10: 181–185

Jarvis P 1985 The sociology of adult and continuing education. Croom Helm, London.

Johns CC 1993 Guided reflection. In: Palmer A, Burns S, Bulman C (eds) Reflective practice in nursing: growth of the professional practitioner. Blackwell Scientific, Oxford

Jones RG 1990 The lecture as a teaching method in modern nurse education. Nurse Education Today 10: 290–293

Kenworthy N, Nicklin P 1988 Teaching and assessing in nursing practice. An experiential approach. Scutari Press, London

Knowles M 1990 The adult learner: a neglected species. Gulf Publishing, London

Lauterbach S, Hentz-Becker P 1996 Caring for self: becoming a self reflective nurse. Holistic Nursing Practice 10: 57–68

Mezirow J 1981 A critical theory for adult learning and education. Adult Education 32: 3–24

Nielson BB 1992 Applying androgogy in nursing continuing education. Journal of Continuing Education in Nursing 23: 148–151

O'Kell SP 1988 A study of the relationships between learning style, readiness for self-directed learning and teacher preference in one health district. Nurse Education Today 8: 197–204

Powell JH 1989 The reflective practitioner in nursing. Journal of Advanced Nursing 14: 824–832

Quality Assurance Agency 2004 Guidelines on the accreditation of prior learning. Draft for consultation – February. QAA, London, p. 3. On-line at: http://www.qaa.ac.uk/public/apel/draft/guidance.htm. Accessed March 29 2004

Quinn F 1995 The principles and practice of nurse education. Croom Helm, London

Reece I, Walker S 1995 A practical guide to teaching, training and learning, 2nd edn. Business Education Publishers Limited, Sunderland

Rolfe G 1997 Beyond expertise: theory, practice and the reflexive practitioner. Journal of Clinical Nursing 6: 93–97

Rolfe G, Freshwater D, Jasper M 2001 Critical reflection for nursing and the helping professions; a user's guide. Palgrave, Basingstoke

Rowntree D 1987 Assessing students: how shall we know them? Kogan Page, London

Schon D 1991 The reflective practitioner: how professionals think in action. Avebury: Aldershot

SECC 2003 Credit level descriptors for further and higher education. Southern England Consortium for Credit Accumulation and Transfer, London

Steinaker N, Bell M 1979 The experiential taxonomy: a new approach to teaching and learning. Academic Press, New York

Street A 1991 From image to action – reflection in nursing practice. Deakin University, Geelong

United Kingdom Central Council for Nursing, Midwifery and Health Visiting 1992 Code of professional conduct for the nurse, midwife and health visitor. UKCC, London

United Kingdom Central Council for Nursing, Midwifery and Health Visiting 1999a Fitness for practice. The UKCC Commission for Nursing and Midwifery Education (Chair: Sir Leonard Peach). UKCC, London

United Kingdom Central Council for Nursing, Midwifery and Health Visiting 1999b UKCC PREP monitor project: summary report. UKCC, London

While A 1994 Competence versus performance, which is more important? Journal of Advanced Nursing 20: 525–531

Useful websites

Council of Deans: www.councilofdeans.org.uk/docs/breaking/htm

Deliberations on Teaching and Learning in Higher Education: www.city.londonmet.ac.uk/deliberations/

Institution of Learning and Teaching in Higher Education: www.ilt.ac.uk

Nursing and Midwifery Council: www.nmc-uk.org

14 Getting the most from practice learning

Maggie Mallik

INTRODUCTION

Practice placements are the most stimulating areas for learning on a professional healthcare course. Students state they learn not only patient/client care but also about themselves and their personal development. Time spent in placement learning is very demanding psychologically, emotionally, and physically but has potential for great satisfaction. As an adult learner whether in nursing or midwifery, it is important that you feel involved and in control of your learning experiences. There are many people involved in the process of placement learning. These include:

- you, the student of midwifery or nursing
- the patient/client in all areas where you will be placed to gain your learning experiences
- those members of the health and social care teams who are providing for patient/client care and who will become involved in supporting, supervising and assessing your learning
- the university team who organize your course and provide advice and personal tutorial support.

The aim of this chapter is to provide you with insight into and practical hints on how to get the most out of the experience of learning in a practice environment.

GAINING INSIGHT TO THE PRACTICE LEARNING ENVIRONMENT

Practice placement experience is an integral part of any course that prepares you for a professional qualification as well as an academic award. The total amount of time spent in practice settings during the course is a statutory requirement if you are to register to practice in your chosen profession. What may differ between courses is:

- the organization and timing of when practice placements occur
- the type of placement selected to meet the learning outcomes of the course
- the amount of time spent in each placement
- the specific learning outcomes/competencies to be achieved in each placement.

In providing health care, your placement could be a residential unit and/or nursing home in the community, a ward area or a specialist unit in an acute hospital, working with an individual practitioner or a team in providing nursing and midwifery care in the home or in a primary care setting. Overall the aim of providing a variety of placement areas for learning is to enable you to 'identify the community focus of care, the continuing nature of care, the need for acute and critical care and the multi-professional approach to care' (Royal College of Nursing, 2002, p. 2).

What is important for you to understand is that learning in a practice placement is a completely different experience from learning in an academic setting.

Learning in an academic setting has been likened to learning 'in an ivory tower' when compared with learning 'in the swampy lowlands' of practice. What images do these 'quotes' conjure up in your mind?

It may be that these 'quotes' present contradictory images for you, depending on what you view as important for your progress to becoming a healthcare professional. The 'ivory tower' of university classroom learning may be deemed as high up in the hierarchy of learning, and also as safe and secure. It also could be seen as being isolated from what the healthcare professional really needs to know in order to 'do the job'. The 'swampy lowlands' may conjure up an image of risk and danger, an unpredictable place where unexpected things happen. In this environment the individual needs to have considerable skills and knowledge to negotiate 'the swamps' and to become competent in dealing with uncertainty. However, the challenge in learning to be a safe practitioner in 'the lowlands' produces its own satisfaction and rewards.

Researchers who have studied the issues that affect students' learning in the practice setting refer to the existence of 'a practice-learning environment'. Factors that may affect this learning environment and have the potential to make it a positive or a negative experience for the student include the:

- behaviour and influence of the placement leader
- attitudes of the practice team to learners
- nature of the relationship between the learner and practice mentor/assessor
- confidence and teaching ability of the mentor/assessor
- type of patients/clients who receive care and/or treatment
- physical, psychological and emotional workload
- amount and type of support available
- organization and implementation of teaching and assessing
- congruence between theory and practice to include the relationship between the area and the academic institution.

All these factors will interact and may, in the ideal situation, provide for an environment that is highly supportive of your learning in a particular placement. Some negative experiences can be counterbalanced by more positive structures to create a balanced environment. You also have to be aware that there may be strong negative influences that are difficult to change and you may need extra help and resources to deal with these. In your course, you are going to have experience in a broad spectrum of practice placements with their respective learning environments.

Keep and record your descriptions, feelings, reactions and responses in your reflective diary. This will help you to analyse on how you have coped with each of the different situations you have met. More importantly, it will allow you to monitor your own personal and professional development through learning from those experiences (see Chapters 11 and 13).

There are websites where students exchange their reactions and feelings about their practice experiences or gain insight through exchanging information: see http://www.student-nurse.fsnet.co.uk/ for nurses and http://studentmidwives.co.uk/ for student midwives.

It is important to read the following case study and the analysis that follows as it illustrates some of the factors that can affect your learning while in a practice placement.

Samara, a mature student, was on her first placement in an adult ward that dealt with patients with acute medical conditions. It was her fourth week of a 10-week placement and she was at last beginning to feel at home in the ward. She had worked hard in completing any tasks that were set on each shift. Samara had been described as 'a good student' by the practice team. She also had a good relationship with her mentor and she had even been asked out by members of the team to a ward 'night out' for a member of staff who was leaving. She was satisfied and told her husband how much she was enjoying the learning experience.

John was an elderly man who had been admitted to the ward with a mild stroke 5 days ago. Samara had been given some responsibility for his care by her mentor and had developed a good relationship with John. She felt that he trusted her and that her care and encouragement had made a difference to his wellbeing and ability to recover from the stroke. John was ready for discharge and was looking forward to going home.

On the morning of discharge, John's condition suddenly deteriorated and he collapsed while in the toilet. The cardiac arrest team were called and Samara felt helpless and anxious during the subsequent resuscitation attempt, which was unsuccessful. Other members of staff, including Samara's mentor, did not have time to give her any extra support following the incident. Samara finished her shift feeling upset, tired, frightened and alone. She was unable to talk to her mentor and she later offloaded her worries to her husband.

The following day Samara did have a chance to sit and talk with her mentor, who was able to go through her feelings with her but also encouraged her to write the incident down in her reflective diary and try to learn from what had happened.

Samara's story illustrates a number of key issues about the complex nature of the practice area as an environment for learning. Although Samara was a mature adult with life experience, she recognized her place and role as a student. Practice placements can have a hierarchy and it is important to learn where you fit into this hierarchy. As a student you are a transient member of the team and much depends on how students are viewed and accepted by the placement team. At the beginning of the placement, students should concentrate on being able to 'fit in' with the team and 'do the work' that is required. In our story, Samara had perceived that this goal was necessary; she had achieved this goal and was accepted by the team.

Practice placements do present you with a challenge of how to cope with unexpected and unpredictable happenings. They are risky places to work. You can be made to feel safe by the support of the practice team, and in particular an understanding mentor who learns more about your fears and worries than other members of the team. Samara had built up a good relationship with her mentor and was beginning to feel safe by her fourth week in the area.

You can feel pressurized by the need to perform in front of others. When she was given responsibilities that she could deal with competently, Samara felt she was doing well. However, when John collapsed, at this stage of her course she did not have the skills to contribute much to the resuscitation effort. She needed to come to terms with the fact that this was acceptable for her level of experience, but no one had time to reinforce that with her. You need to recognize that practice areas are a place of public performance but you need to be secure in what you are capable of doing and not expect too much from yourself.

Samara needed reassurance, support and teaching about the situation she had just witnessed but the team was too busy dealing with the situation at the time. Events can happen that will mean your need for support and your learning priorities are in competition with patient care needs. This requires you to be sensitive and recognize the priorities of staff in the area and not to be offended if your needs seem to be ignored or are low down in the hierarchy of needs to be dealt with at the time. Her mentor dealt with Samara's needs on the following day when there was less pressure on her time to provide patient care. Samara used another method of coping in being able to talk through her experience with her husband. Using your peer group for support is equally valid.

Samara was tired, anxious and upset by John's sudden death. She illustrates that working in a healthcare placement can demand a lot of psychological and emotional labour as well as the physical doing of the work. You can expect to feel very tired and unable to participate in your social life as fully as you would be doing when attending lectures. However, as you learn from the experience and begin to cope with the unexpected, the feeling of satisfaction and enjoyment will act as a powerful motivator to continue your learning from practice experience.

Although the above example reflects an experience that might happen in an acute hospital placement, there are parallel situations; whether you are a midwifery student who might have to deal with an emergency situation when a mother is in labour; or a mental health branch student where a patient suddenly becomes aggressive and attention seeking; or a child branch student where parents are having difficulty coping with their child's injuries after a playground accident; or a student caring for those with learning disabilities coping with the sudden out-of-control behaviours of a teenager who fears strangers in their environment. For any situation that causes you stress, try to debrief as soon as possible after the event so that you can reflect on the situation and with the help of your mentor turn it into a positive learning experience.

PREPARING FOR YOUR PRACTICE PLACEMENT

During your course you will be allocated to a broad range of practice placement areas. The sequence in which you are allocated will have been worked out to suit the academic programme you are following on the course.

As a midwifery student your placements might be organized around a caseload model so you might be allocated to a team of midwives who are responsible for the care of a set allocation of pregnant women. Most midwifery practice takes place in the community setting. If you are completing a course in mental health nursing you may be expected to gain insight and experience by caring for a person with a mental health problem who is coping with living at home or in a community unit. On an adult nursing course you may be studying a unit or module of learning on the healthcare needs of elderly people and your next placement is matched to this. It might be an allocation to a nursing home setting for the elderly or a day hospital or an acute elderly care unit.

A specialist module or even special preparation for practice sessions may be organized in order to prepare you for the learning experience. Most universities also supply you with a booklet outlining the objectives, opportunities and regulations for practice learning. The Royal College of Nursing has recently produced a 'toolkit' document, which is helpful especially in outlining the value of placement learning and your role in ensuring that you gain the most from your experiences (Royal College of Nursing 2002). However, sometimes the sequencing of practice placement areas is not so neat and tidy and you may have received some theoretical input related to a particular client group several months prior to meeting that group in a placement area.

Much of the material you learn on your academic course may be delivered to you as subject knowledge, for example in sessions on biological and/or the psychosocial sciences. It may be up to you as the student to select the knowledge you need from each of these subject areas in order to help you understand a particular practice experience.

Having found out some information about your next practice placement, reflect on what specific areas of subject knowledge might be useful for you to revise in order to prepare yourself for giving care to the specific patient/client group.

Placements for healthcare courses can be spread over a large geographical area, sometimes with a mixture of allocation to practice placements in the town and/or the countryside. You may be allocated to what is known as a 'home (NHS) trust'. This means that for the whole of your course you will be allocated to a mixture of placements in the acute hospital and community area in one specific locality, e.g. a district hospital, a nearby primary care (NHS) trust and local community health and social care teams, GP practices and private hospitals. Many 'home trusts' take an active interest in the particular group of students allocated to them and often organize a specific full-day orientation programme for the total student group at the beginning of the course. The Trust education support team takes responsibility for ensuring you:

- know the main layout of the Trust
- gain access to Trust premises through obtaining staff identity cards
- can access their library and other learning facilities such as practice learning and e-learning centres if available
- register to use their computers
- are measured for uniforms and obtain these if needed for your practice placement experiences
- are aware of who to contact for additional learning support, e.g. the Clinical Placement Facilitator (CPF)/practice educators (PEs)/ lecturer practitioners (LPs)/link lecturers (LLs) and where they are based within the Trust and the local health community
- visit areas and meet key members of teams that are particularly relevant to your programme; e.g. midwifery students will meet the core team and visit appropriate practice areas.

Most NHS trusts have extensive staff development facilities, which reflects their commitment to a strategy for 'lifelong learning' (Department of Health 2000) for all their staff. Many, through their partnerships with local universities and colleges, employ education personnel who have a responsibility to ensure a good learning environment for all learners accessing placements within the Trust. A key person for providing support for nursing and midwifery students will be the Clinical Placement Facilitator (CPF). This person may have a team of 'practice educators' (PEs) working with them to provide support in particular areas across the 'home trust' site.

Accommodation may be offered to students on hospital sites as an alternative to staying on the university campus. Regardless of where you may be living there will always be the need to travel to and from the university and/or the placement sites. Ensure you know what you are entitled to claim for reimbursement of travel, as these expenses are often an added burden when trying to cope with the limited funds you have as a student.

- Most NHS trusts now have web sites where you can access information on the Trust and its activities. Many contain information accessible to the public on each of their ward and unit areas and specialist services. This is a quick and easy way to gain insight and information.
- Many universities have also negotiated through their partnerships with NHS placement areas to post information on placements on their own student information websites. Check out whether this is available in your university.

It is important to learn as much as possible about the client groups that you are going to be working with in the practice setting. Sometimes, your preparation time is limited and/or the material presented in academic sessions is broad and generic and not specific enough to your learning needs for a particular placement. Fellow students or those more senior to you often provide the more detailed information you need, especially if they have just completed time in the area. Increasingly, students are using the 'chat rooms' on websites to exchange information about practice placement areas and types (see annotated websites).

Be aware that 'stories' about placement experiences can be embellished, so try to maintain an open mind and focus on the specific information that you feel would be helpful to you. Remember that preparation time is limited so do not expect to achieve too much. The university performs an education audit of all placement areas and passes them as suitable for your learning. This means that the practice area will often have the resources to provide you with additional focused learning material and opportunities when you start on the placement.

During specific time set aside to prepare for placement try to find out the following:

- How will knowledge and skills that I have learned in the past be transferable to this practice placement?
- What specific knowledge and skills would be helpful for coping with learning in the particular practice placement?
- Are there any clinical skills that I might need to practice in the safe environment of the school's skills laboratory? Arrange time to practice these skills.
- How are practice placement staff informed about my stage on the course and my capabilities?
- What sort of commitment is expected or should be expected from me in terms of shifts, doing night duty or weekend work?

There are formal rules governing the amount of time you spend in your practice placement. On a professional nursing/midwifery course, this time is specified by the registration board (the Nursing and Midwifery Council (NMC) in the UK) and then organized by the university to fit within your course structure. Attendance during your practice placement is carefully monitored and a set number of hours must be completed before you will be allowed to register as a nurse or midwife. The registration board also recommends the broad categories of placement you complete and these will generally fit the requirements set down locally and by other countries, such as those within the European Union. This means that, once registered, your qualification is accepted (with some reservations) if you wish to work as a registered practitioner elsewhere in the world.

The length of time in each placement area should be sufficient for you to achieve your learning outcomes and the competencies required for your stage of training. Patterns of time do vary, to include a mixture of shorter 4/6-week placements up to longer periods of 12 weeks in one area just prior to completing your programme. Some placement experiences have been organized around a 'learning circuit model'/'hub and spoke model' in which, during a practice placement in one area, you complete shorter observational visits to areas that link with the 'hub ward'. These 'spokes' allow you to observe specialist input and continuity in the care of patients/clients.

Sometimes you may have control of the placement through undertaking a mapping of a specific 'patient/client journey' through the healthcare system with the concurrent completion of a case study for inclusion in your portfolio of practice learning. In midwifery, this latter model is a dominant feature, as taking on a supervised caseload of 'mothers to be' is the most common feature of learning to be a midwife. Much of the practice learning related to caring for those with a learning disability and with mental health problems also follows a caseload approach.

Many universities also offer the opportunity to do an 'elective placement' where you can choose an area for gaining practice experience. This could be undertaken anywhere in the world provided that it is carefully organized and that learning outcomes can be achieved.

Understanding supernumerary status

Students undergoing a practice placement are agreed to have what is termed 'supernumerary status' within the working team. You should be aware that there are many different ways in which supernumerary status is interpreted in practice. In the past students were paid a salary while undertaking training and were counted as an essential part of the working team. This meant that wards and units had to have a set number of students allocated to their area in order to provide the service to patients. The learning needs of students were often considered to be secondary to the work needs of the placement.

Although learning through working is legitimate and is still considered an important part of your placement experience, because of the change to 'supernumerary status' students are not now counted as an integral part of the workforce. In theory, this means that your placement area should not count on you being there as essential to provide the service to patients. You should not be expected to work the same shifts as the permanent contracted staff in the area and if there is opportunity to follow up a specific learning situation you should be enabled to do so.

In reality, many students choose to work the same shift pattern as their mentors in order to be supported consistently by the same person. Some practice areas feel that by working the same shifts as the permanent staff you gain experience and insight into the demands of your future role as a qualified nurse or midwife. This is considered part of the socialization process into the culture of health care and the particular profession you aspire to join (Lave and Wenger 1991).

Many areas are flexible and will allow students to negotiate their time in placements. However, you should be aware that the start time of any shift is important for an organized handover of information and most areas will expect students to commence the shift at the same time as the practice team. Good timekeeping is a key issue for practice staff and it is noted very quickly if a student makes a habit of arriving late for the shift.

As a student, you should be considered as 'supernumerary' to the team. However as you become a more senior student, during your third year, you may be expected to gain experience by completing all shift patterns, including weekend work and night duty. This longer time in a practice placement gives you insight to the experience of working full time as a registered nurse or midwife once you have completed your studies.

The following is a list of practical things to do once your practice placement area has been named:

- Find out the key contact name and phone number and ring that person to arrange a preliminary visit
- Ensure that you know the name and telephone contact number of the CPF/PE and/or the university lecturer who links with the area
- Check on how to get to the placement and how much time needs to be set aside for travelling
- Ensure that you know the cost of travelling and how to claim for reimbursement if it is available.

Making the initial contact with the placement

Your placement allocation office should provide you with the name of your area, a contact name and number and a brief outline on how to get to your placement. Although all arrangements have been made in advance, it is still possible for students to turn up on the first day of their placement time and find that the area staff are not expecting them. It is important, therefore, that you ring the placement prior to the start date. The contact name is likely to be the supervising midwife for the unit, your specific allocated midwife or the clinical manager for the area of practice. You may then be informed as to who has been specifically allocated from the team to support you during your placement. There are many titles used for this person, e.g. mentor, assessor, practice supervisor. The most common term used in nursing and midwifery is 'mentor' (Department of Health and English National Board 2001).

Some units will welcome you visiting the area prior to your start date. Others may not like you to visit and indicate that they have a special orientation programme prepared for you on your first day. The LL or LP might provide this, or the area may have a member of staff, e.g. a practice development nurse or practice educator, who is responsible for the orientation of all new staff. Besides introducing yourself to the key contact for the area, the following list of activities are things to do on that first visit to your practice placement.

- Give the staff information on the stage of your training and cross-check your start date and completion date
- Find out all you need to know regarding shifts; what is expected of you; what the start and completion times of shifts are; what shift you will be working on the first day
- Check who will be your mentor and, if possible, meet them
- Negotiate any key off-duty arrangements that you might need
- Check whether you need to wear a uniform or not. Does the area have any special dress codes if you are not required to wear a uniform?
- Check-out arrangements for catering if you are on long shifts – is there a canteen, staff room, fridge for your own refreshments?
- Locate where to hang your coat and store your valuables

INITIATING THE PRACTICE LEARNING EXPERIENCE

Up to now we have concentrated on giving you some insight into the practice learning environment and how to prepare yourself for your experience in your practice placement. Although your first placement is a key event in your career, every placement is unique and special. In time, when you have built up a repertoire of skills, you cope more easily with change. The following sections will give you some advice on how to deal with the actual experience itself.

Getting through the first day

Most students feel nervous and anxious about their first day in a new placement, even more so if it is their first placement on the course. If you have done your preparation well then some of that nervous energy can be directed into getting to know the team and your surroundings on the first day. Do not be hard on yourself or the placement staff. The first day in any new environment is stressful, whether you are a student or not, so just try to 'fit in'. It is a unique experience for you but the staff may be used to having a new batch of students start in their area at frequent intervals so it may not be a special occasion for them.

Remember that you are not required to know everything after the first day, or even after the first week. Be prepared for some of the issues indicated in the section on dealing with the practice environment. Expect to feel very tired and emotionally drained at the end of the day.

Some areas will have an induction programme set up for you and will take you through that in an organized way. This is helpful and more cost-effective if a number of students are starting on the same day. Other areas may require you to join a member of the team and become involved in the daily work as soon as you start. This may seem daunting at first but, provided you are closely supervised, will give you a feeling of satisfaction at the end of the day. You may be attached to an individual practitioner such as a community midwife or a community psychiatric nurse, in which case you may feel much less isolated and more supported on your first day. However, work on building a rapport with your mentor will be important and can take up a considerable amount of emotional energy on the first day.

Regardless of whether there is an induction programme, your mentor or a member of the team should ensure that you are given information on key health and safety features within the area during the first day. These features include:

- emergency numbers for fire and the cardiac arrest team
- location of fire fighting equipment and exits
- location of the cardiac arrest equipment (if appropriate)
- preliminary information and guidance on any health and safety issue that is a particular feature of the practice location.

Try to clarify what will be expected of you, as a student, should any emergency situation arise. Some practice areas provide a 'checklist' to indicate that you have been informed of these health and safety guidelines and may assess your knowledge of the procedures later in your placement. Mentors will also check that you have received the statutory moving and handling training before allowing you to move loads and/or patients/clients.

- Make sure you are on time and introduce yourself to the person in charge of the team
- If you are not allocated to be supervised by a particular individual, try to attach yourself to someone in the team
- Participate as much as you can – actually doing something will make you feel better than just standing and observing

Writing your personal learning objectives

Consider the first week as an orientation period when you are concentrating on getting to know the place, the people and the patients/clients. Do not insist on the first day that you have certain personal learning objectives to achieve and demand to know how the practice team is going to help you achieve them. Unless requested from you, discussion of your objectives can wait until the end of the first week; you may then need to take the initiative in setting up a preliminary interview with your mentor. Being assertive with the right approach is important in achieving your goals.

Prior to the experience you should discuss your objectives with your personal tutor and/or module leader. These may be related to the competencies that need to be assessed and/or to any theoretical work that is being completed alongside the placement experience. Evaluation of your previous experience may highlight key areas that you need to develop further. Some of these competencies may be very important to achieve in order for you to progress to another stage of your course. Many areas can provide you with an orientation booklet that also includes a list of objectives the practice team feels you should be able to achieve because of the experience available.

Some objectives can be written before a placement, especially if it is a short observational visit. These are very helpful for the person who is looking after you as they can structure the short time available to achieve the objectives. For longer placements, setting and discussing the learning outcomes at the beginning ensures that evaluation of the degree of their achievement is much more productive during the intermediate and final interviews of the placement.

Do not expect too much from yourself or the practice placement. You have to find out how the personal objectives you have might match up with what is actually on offer in the placement. There will also be competencies that you have to achieve. Find out if they can be achieved easily or whether special arrangements need to be made for you to practise a particular skill. You need to take responsibility for reminding people or negotiating on the spot if that experience becomes available unexpectedly.

Complete the following activities prior to first interview:

■ List the areas of care in which you wish to have more practice

■ Check your assessment document – there may be certain competencies that you must achieve in this placement

■ Note in the first week what type of experience is available in the area and prepare to discuss with your mentor how this experience will help you achieve your objectives

NEGOTIATING THE MENTOR–STUDENT RELATIONSHIP

Most if not all practice placements will allocate a named member of the healthcare team to act as your support and guide while on the placement. As stated earlier in the chapter, your placement area may use the terms 'mentor', 'preceptor', 'assessor' and 'practice supervisor' interchangeably, depending on the placement context and the assumed meanings ascribed to the role. The most common term is 'mentor'. Some areas may also allocate a second named mentor as a 'back-up' person to cover for times when your named mentor is not available because of annual leave, night duty or days off. This person is sometimes known as an 'associate mentor'. In most instances, your mentor will also be your assessor and will complete all activities related to the assessment of your learning in practice.

■ On your preplacement visit, find out what is the normal way of organizing support for you in the area

■ Get to know the name of your 'mentor' and meet them if possible

■ Request that you work the same shift as your mentor, particularly during your first week in the area

■ If allocated an 'associate mentor', clarify how they will help you and the processes involved in completing your practice assessment

If your practice placement area allows you to do your own off duty, ensure that you negotiate with your mentor how often you should work together. Although it is important that you get consistent support from the same person at the beginning of your placement, it may also be helpful to have a break from each other. Working with other people within the team allows you to observe and reflect on different approaches to care and to develop your skills in building new working relationships. This break in observing how you work and learn will also allow your mentor to more easily assess the degree of progress you are making. In community placements, when allocated to work with a specific practitioner such as a midwife, district nurse or community psychiatric nurse, they will often organize set periods to work with other members of the multiprofessional team to include those involved in social care.

You and your mentor should meet together as soon as possible after you start in your placement. Your initial time together may be very focused on your orientation and helping you to settle in and getting to know the physical layout and the 'routines' of the area or the practice case load (community placements). It is also important that you both try to make time at the end of the shift to sit in a quiet place with the aim of getting to know one another and the expectations you each have of your time in the placement. Do not be surprised if your contact in the first week is kept at an informal level, as this is an important time in building up your personal relationship separate from negotiating the more formal professional relationship inherent in the 'assessor' role.

At your initial formal meeting (which will be called the first or preliminary interview in the assessment documentation), it will be important for both of you to review and complete your assessment documentation and your learning objectives for your time in the placement. You both need to check out your individual interpretations of what knowledge and skills you bring to the placement and the areas where you need the most support and guidance in order to successfully achieve the learning outcomes and the required level of competence.

■ In some areas, ensuring that you and your mentor work together may not be a high priority for the staff. You may have to be more proactive and assertive in ensuring that you have an allocated mentor and that you work together and reflect on your progress at key times during your placement. In community placements this is not usually an issue as you are usually working on a one-to-one basis with your mentor.

- If you have difficulties, discuss these as soon as possible with the person in charge of the placement and/or your CPF/PE or the Link Lecturer from the university.

- When you have completed your first formal interview, ensure that you arrange, at that time, a date for your intermediate/mid-placement meeting.

Facilitating feedback

Your first interview is a key time to negotiate when you and your mentor should work together and when you should meet for formal progress feedback sessions. It is important not to underestimate the difficulties that might arise in making these arrangements. Problems usually centre on the mentor being unavailable when you are in the placement. If your shift pattern is different from those in the practice area, more problems arise in accommodating working together and meetings. Your mentor may be completing 12-hour shifts when you are doing 7.5 hours per day. This means the mentor will be working fewer days in the week than you are. The mentor may be doing internal rotation on to night duty and, unless you negotiate to do night duty alongside them, they will not be available for sometimes up to 2 weeks because of having 'nights off'. As a student, you may not be required or may not wish to work over the weekends, again limiting the time you will work together.

Most practice assessment documentation requires that you have a formal interview with your mentor half way through your time in placement. This is known as the 'intermediate' interview and is a very important stage as this is a key time to receive constructive feedback on your progress. It then allows you time to develop and improve on your current abilities in order to achieve your competencies at the required level by the end of the placement. If your time in the placement is short, it can be difficult to arrange this interview time with your mentor. However, it is important to make the effort to ensure formal feedback on your progress from a member of the practice team, for example your 'associate' mentor if your allocated mentor is not available. It is also an opportunity to have competencies and achievements (such as portfolio evidence) signed off.

Your final interview with your mentor is very important to review the completion of your assessment documentation and the achievement of your learning objectives. It is very inconvenient for both you and the mentor if you have to return to a placement area after you have completed your time. Try to ensure that you meet your mentor at the beginning of the last week in placement so that if the session is postponed there will still be time before you leave the practice setting.

■ Keep a record of activities that you feel have helped you achieve your competencies and use these to remind your mentor at the intermediate and final interviews

■ If at all possible, ask for daily feedback. The following prompt questions can be asked:
  – How do you think I got on today?
  – What did I do well?
  – What could I improve on?
  – What did I leave out?

■ Record your daily experiences and mentor feedback in your reflective diary

Dealing with problems

Sometimes it does happen that a student and mentor are unable to form a productive professional relationship for mutual support and learning because they just do not like each other at a personal level. When this happens in our lives, we usually make choices and avoid any contact with the person. However, in a practice placement, feeling that you wish to avoid your mentor will have an obvious detrimental effect on your learning in that area. The situation needs to be dealt with as early, as honestly and as sensitively as possible. It may be that you choose to resolve this problem yourself or that you ask for help from the CPF/PE/LL. Resolving the issue is even more important if you are in the area for a substantial length of time, there is no 'associate' mentor, and/or when you and the mentor have to work very closely together on a one-to-one basis, as in community placements.

Most universities have guidelines in place that will steer you through what to do if you have problems while on practice placements. These are very important if there are concerns regarding your competence and ability to achieve your learning outcomes by the end of your placement experience (see Chapter 6).

■ *Consider what sort of feedback you find helpful in motivating you to learn and perform better in your role*

■ *Remember that your mentor may also be learning the role of mentor and may wish to have some feedback from you*

■ *Giving each other mutual feedback that is positive will improve and enhance your working relationship*

MAKING PROGRESS IN YOUR PLACEMENT

Compared to the experience of learning in the classroom, practice placements offer an infinite variety of encounters for learning. It is helpful to isolate some aspects of this learning in order to help you negotiate the 'swampy lowlands'.

Practising clinical skills on patients/clients

A component of your practice assessment is being able to perform physical assessment and physical care skills safely. Students can be very preoccupied during their early weeks in placements with getting to know the staff and being able to do the work. 'Doing the work' involves the mastery of practice-based skills. Initially, students are concerned about their own inadequacy and are frightened of making errors, particularly if the patient/client could suffer as a result of those errors. These fears may make you feel cautious about undertaking practice skills.

Practice skills may be core skills in assessing the healthcare needs of patient/clients. For the student midwife, assessing the gestation period accurately is a core skill that develops with continuous supervised practice. Providing fundamental care for patients/clients, such as meeting their hygiene, comfort and nutritional needs, is a key element of adult nursing. Skills in communicating effectively and sensitively are essential in healthcare professionals so it is important that you reflect on your interactions with patients/clients in order to improve your abilities. Once mastered in one placement, these skills can be transferred to another placement with no problems or extra learning. Other skills are very specific to the area and you may feel that when you try to practise these skills you have reverted back to being a beginner again (Benner 1984). If you know certain skills are needed in your next placement area and these can be practised in the skills laboratory, in order to give you confidence; take every opportunity to do so before you start on your placement.

Learning a new practice skill can take longer than you think. The practitioner should demonstrate it first and then you should be supervised in carrying out the skill for the first time. Although this might make you feel uncomfortable and sometimes embarrassed, it is important that you do not stand back for too long, but undertake to do the skill. Busy people would rather do 'the job' themselves than supervise you and take twice as long. You need to be assertive if you really want to achieve your objectives. In time, you will be left to perform the skill on your own and as you become more proficient you will become quicker at performing the skill safely.

Y